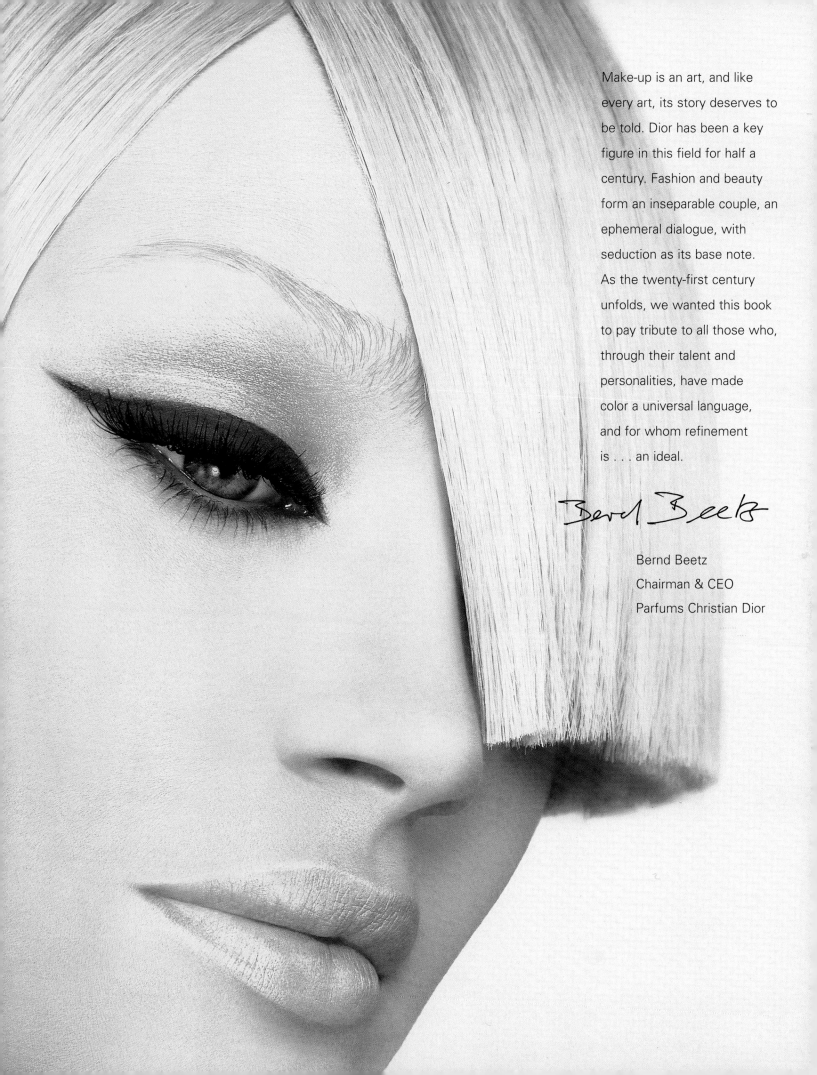

Make-up is an art, and like every art, its story deserves to be told. Dior has been a key figure in this field for half a century. Fashion and beauty form an inseparable couple, an ephemeral dialogue, with seduction as its base note. As the twenty-first century unfolds, we wanted this book to pay tribute to all those who, through their talent and personalities, have made color a universal language, and for whom refinement is . . . an ideal.

Bernd Beetz

Bernd Beetz
Chairman & CEO
Parfums Christian Dior

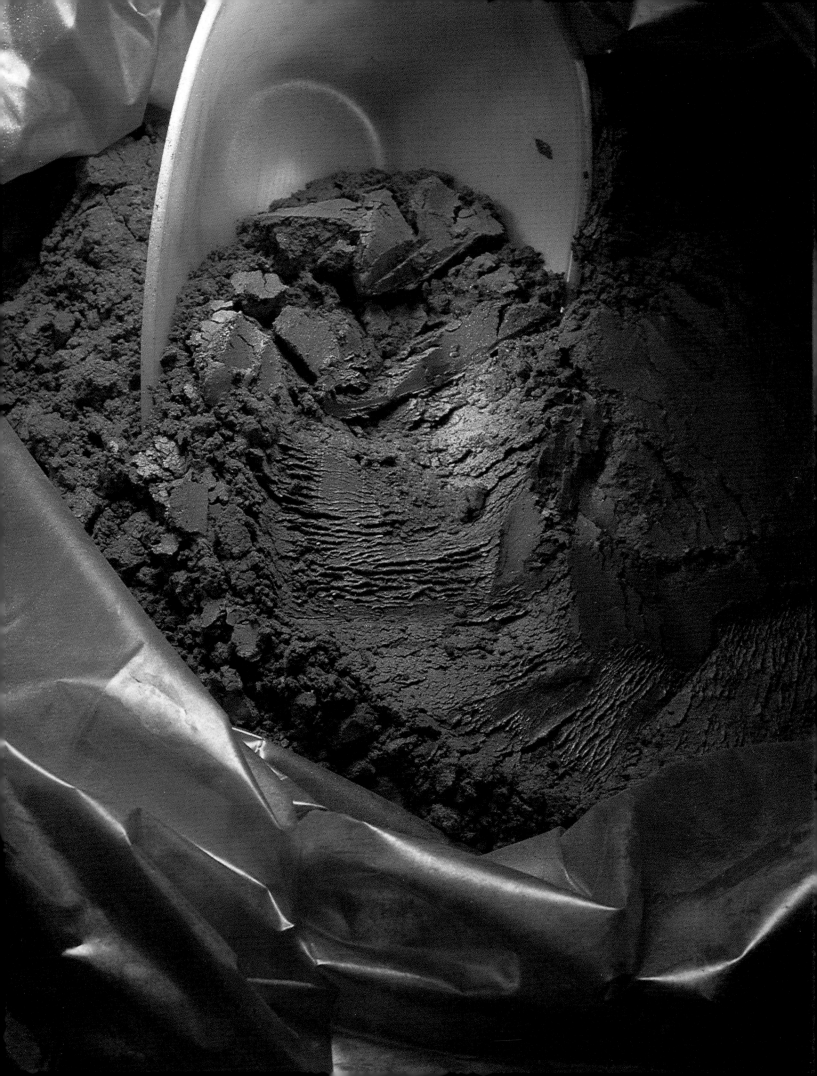

Alain Rustenholz
Make Up

HACHETTE
Illustrated

Acknowledgements

We would like to thank to extend special thanks to Parfums
Christian Dior for their invaluable help. They allowed us to view
their color laboratories and their archives, contributing significantly
to the wealth of illustrations in this book.
Thanks, therefore, to the following people at Parfums
Christian Dior: Tyen, Annie Raynal and Éliane Gouriou, Éliane de la
Béraudière, Sylvie Husson, Julie Wassner and Frédéricke Vance;
Philippe Le Moult and Soizic Pfaff (Christian Dior Couture); Mireille
Sauron, Stéphanie Monnerie and the supervisors for the production
units at Saint-Jean de Braye, where we shot photographs.

Furthermore, we would like to thank all the companies who so
generously provided documentation and illustrations, particularly:
Bourjois (Michèle Duhamel), By Terry (Terry de Gunzburg
and Capucine Juncker), Chanel (Julie Le Blevec), Estée Lauder
(Annie-Claire André), Guerlain (Karine Blanchard), Lancôme
(Françoise de Lapparent), Lanvin (Odile Fraigneau),
Make Up For Ever (Vanessa Lechere), Revlon (Guy Campocasso),
Shiseido (Liliane Ménard and Sonia Mamin), Shu Uemura
(Francine Schlouch).
And finally, we would like to thank Annie Pérez, image and
publications director at the Musée des Arts Décoratifs;
Bertrand Rondot, curator, and his assistant Sophie Motsch, who
allowed us to photograph beauty spot boxes. Special thanks to
Sophie Van der Mey (Lancaster), who gave permission to publish
the photograph taken for Manifesto.

Design and production: Marc Walter / H.M. Éditions
Graphic design: Marc Walter
Photo research and editor: Sabine Arqué-Greenberg
Translator: Lisa Davidson
English copyeditor: Bernard Wooding
Lithography: Ex-Fabrica, Paris

© HM Éditions, 16, rue Camille Pelletan, 92300 Levallois-Perret,
France

This Edition published in 2003 by Hachette Illustrated UK, Octopus
Publishing Group, 2–4 Heron Quays, London, E14 4JP

Printed by Tien Wah, Singapore
ISBN: 1-84430-021-8

p. 1 Duoliner, by Tyen.
p. 2 The Saint-Jean de Braye plant:
mixture of iridescent pigments
(here, cloisonné gold) used
in eyeshadows, powders and
glossy lipsticks.

Contents

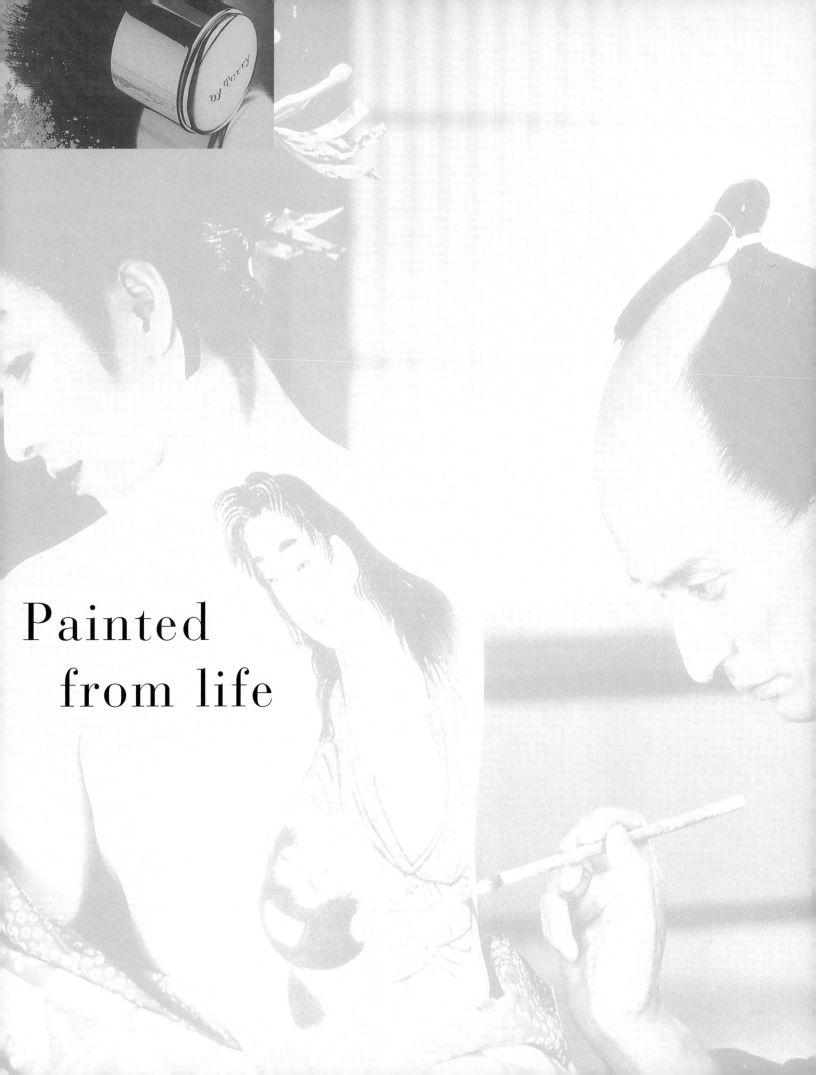

Painted from life

Painted from life

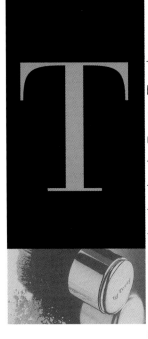

T

The art of painting one's face or body lies somewhere between *trucco*, or artifice in Italian, and make-up, or completion. The first term describes an artistic gesture that considers the face as no more than a support or a surface, while the second expands upon nature by underscoring what already exists: at most, it slightly alters the balance of lines and volumes, shading in one spot to highlight another.

Few ancient writers approved of make-up; Ovid was one who did. For this Greek author, there was no question that culture was better than nature, that human activity improved the natural state of things, that artifice embellished: "Learn, young women, which products enhance your face and by what means you can retain your beauty. Culture forces the most sterile soil to adorn itself with the gifts of Ceres; through it, sharp brambles disappear. Culture sweetens the bitterness of wild fruit, and the grafted tree is improved by its adopted products. Art embellishes everything: marvelous paneling covered with gilding; the earth disappears under marble slabs. More than once, Tyrian purple has been flung in the blazing furnaces, and Indian ivory is sliced into sections to satisfy the refinements of our luxury."

This is how Ovid starts his *Book of Beauty*, before moving on to

"The soul has an indefinable attachment to white; love is happier with red."

Balzac,
La Fille aux yeux d'or

A young Cretan woman (fifteenth century B.C.). Right: Lorenzo Lippi, *Allegory of Simulation* or *The Gardener with a Mask*, ca. 1650, detail. The woman vacillates between the rich red of the pomegranate and the white of the mask. Preceding page: *Five Women Around Utamaro*, film by Kenji Mizoguchi, 1946.

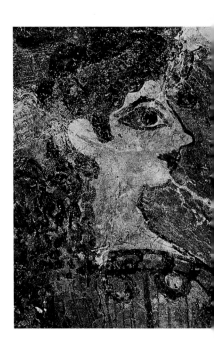

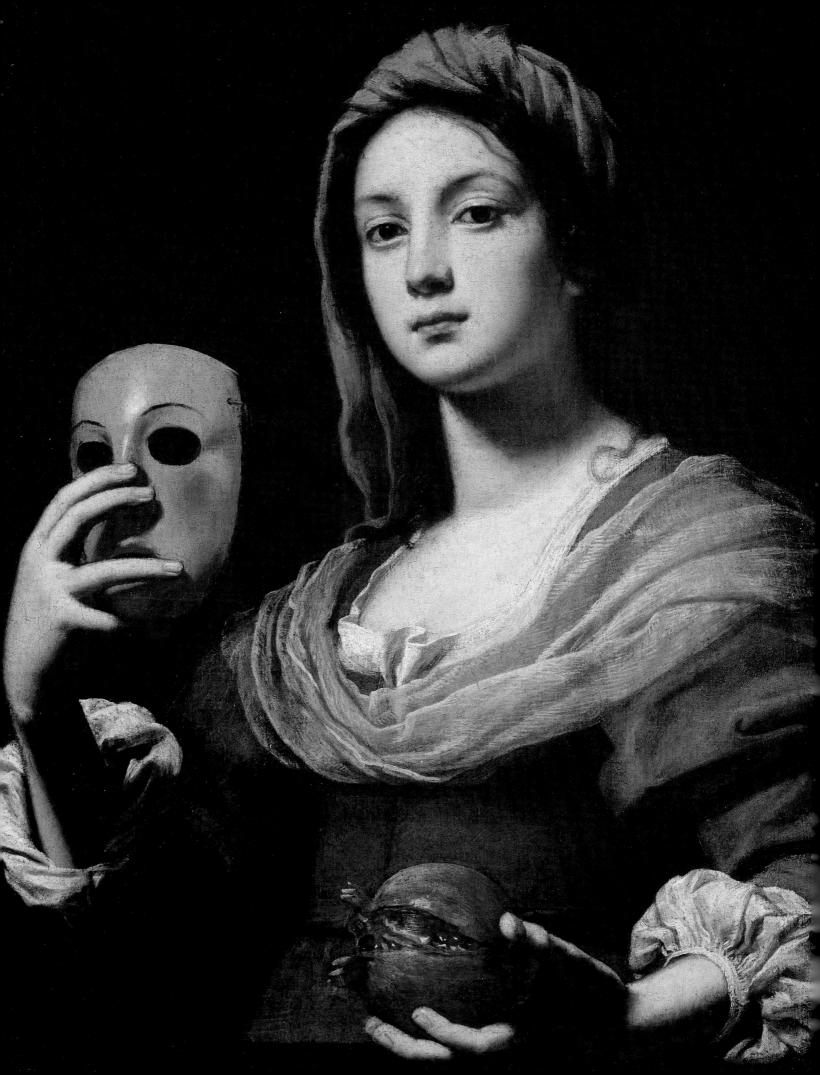

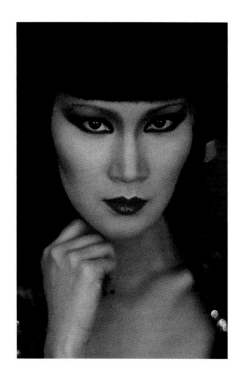

A bright red mouth,
and wide black-rimmed eyes,
accentuated by the make-up
highlighting the Asian features
of this Givenchy model (1990s).

practical advice and recipes. Nearly two thousand years later, Baudelaire made the same choice in favor of culture—probably a poetic choice—by demonstrating an aversion to nature even stronger than Ovid's. "Misfortune to the man, who, like Louis XV, pushes depravation so far as to long for simple nature alone!" he cried. It was for this "natural" penchant that he mocked this king, who had so few ideals and was far more concerned with pursuing worldly pleasures than contemplating beauty. He saw Louis XV as a trivial king who only appreciated women in their simplest possible attire, and only for what he could do with them.

"We know," added Baudelaire, "that when Mme Du Barry wanted to avoid entertaining the king, she was careful to apply rouge. It was a clear enough sign, through which she effectively closed her door. She caused this royal disciple of nature to flee by simply making herself more beautiful."

Does this nature really exist, and if so, where can it be found? Hasn't everything already been modified, improved and arranged by mankind? Indeed, the jet black color of Asian hair, which seems totally natural, was originally supposedly produced by artifice.

In the years during which Baudelaire was writing his *Peintre de la vie moderne*, the Orientalist Stanislas Julien, at the height of his fame, declared to the Institut: "The Chinese knew how to transform and to obtain, using medicines and particular food items, a liquid that would color hair, thereby dying white and red hair to a black color that remained unchanged into old age. This is why the Chinese, by correcting errors of nature, can call themselves 'the black-haired people'."

Nature does make mistakes, art corrects them. This deep black that remains constant from the root of the hair to the tips is not really "natural hair." Would this have been a dye? A dye taken orally, most likely, and therefore more effective and long-lasting than those we use today—in other words, the Chinese would really have been fake brunettes—and since ancient times!

Right: Gianna Maria Canale's
powdered face, doe eyes and
beauty spot in *Mme du Barry*
(Martine Carol played the
leading role), film by
Christian Jaque, 1954.

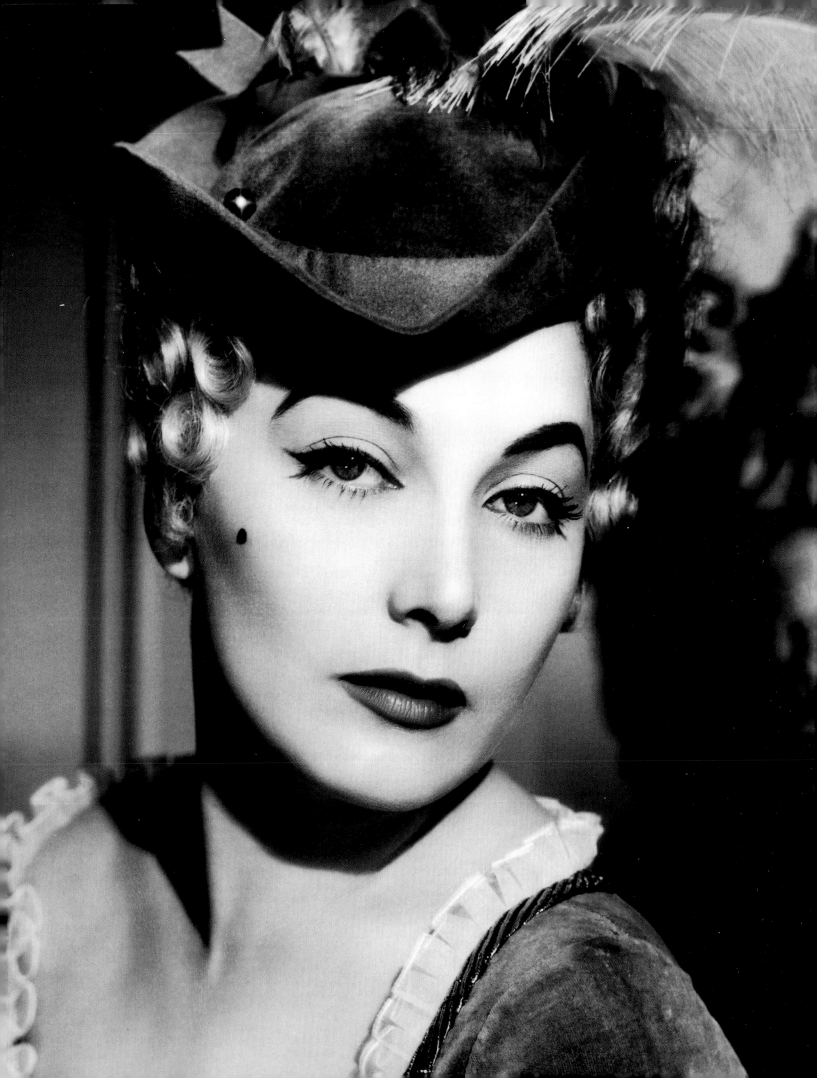

Did it all start with skin care?

Although Stanislas Julien was wrong—and if the Chinese did indeed have this secret, they would no doubt have marketed it by now—this type of explanation was favored over the natural and efficient ones often given for the origin of cosmetics. No sooner had *Homo erectus* started to roam, wandering far from sources of water, than he had to find ways of protecting his skin. Early man understood that metal oxides had anti-bacterial properties, and he mixed them with animal fat; this concoction kept the skin from drying out during long treks.

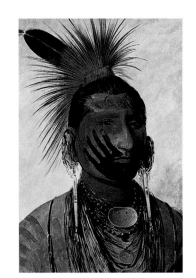

Strong Wind, Chippewa chief by George Catlin, 1845.

Even though Egypt exists as a gift of the Nile River, the days preceding the annual floods were unbearably hot. Flies were everywhere. Needing a way to protect their eyes, Egyptians moistened their eyelids with green make-up, followed by antinomy, which was abundant (in the form of sulfur) along the eastern banks of the Red Sea.

Make-up therefore had a medicinal, preventive purpose, based on necessity. Yet, when examples of eye lotion used for medical purposes were found, dating from 1800 to 1500 B.C., they contained lead, iron, manganese dioxide, copper oxide—though almost never any antinomy. Powdered antinomy sulfide—known in ancient Greece by a word that meant "that which makes the eye large"—seems to have been a beauty product from the start, as opposed to many others, which were purely medicinal.

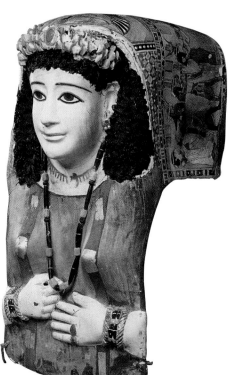

Egyptian mummy mask, Roman era, first century A.D.

The "medical" explanation seems to be much like those at the root of religious food restrictions—the banning of pork, for example—which were based on the highly perishable nature of certain foods in hot climates. Contemporary belief would say that it makes no sense to ban a product if is has no effect, but this is an arbitrary gesture; it exists to define identity, to separate the wheat from the chaff, believers from infidels, civilization from barbarians.

In the same vein, how else can we view cosmetic artifice other than as a specifically human phenomenon, separate from nature and, torn from the primal earth from which the species arose. It affirms that which differentiates us from other kingdoms and is humanity's distinguishing trait. "It was necessary to be painted to be man; he who remained in a state of nature remained indistinguishable from the beasts," wrote Claude Lévi-Strauss about the Brazilian Kaduveo. Earlier, Théophile Gautier had written that "the taste of ornamentation distinguishes the intelligent being from the brute more clearly than any other characteristic. Indeed, no dog has ever dreamed of wearing earrings."

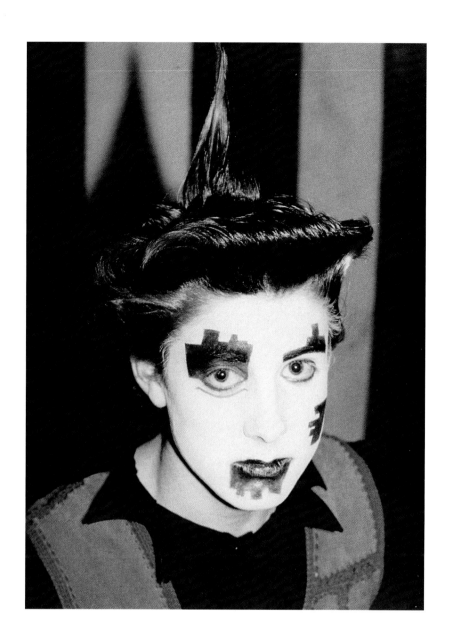

A (de)constructivist style on this decidedly graphic face. Young punk in London, 1990s.

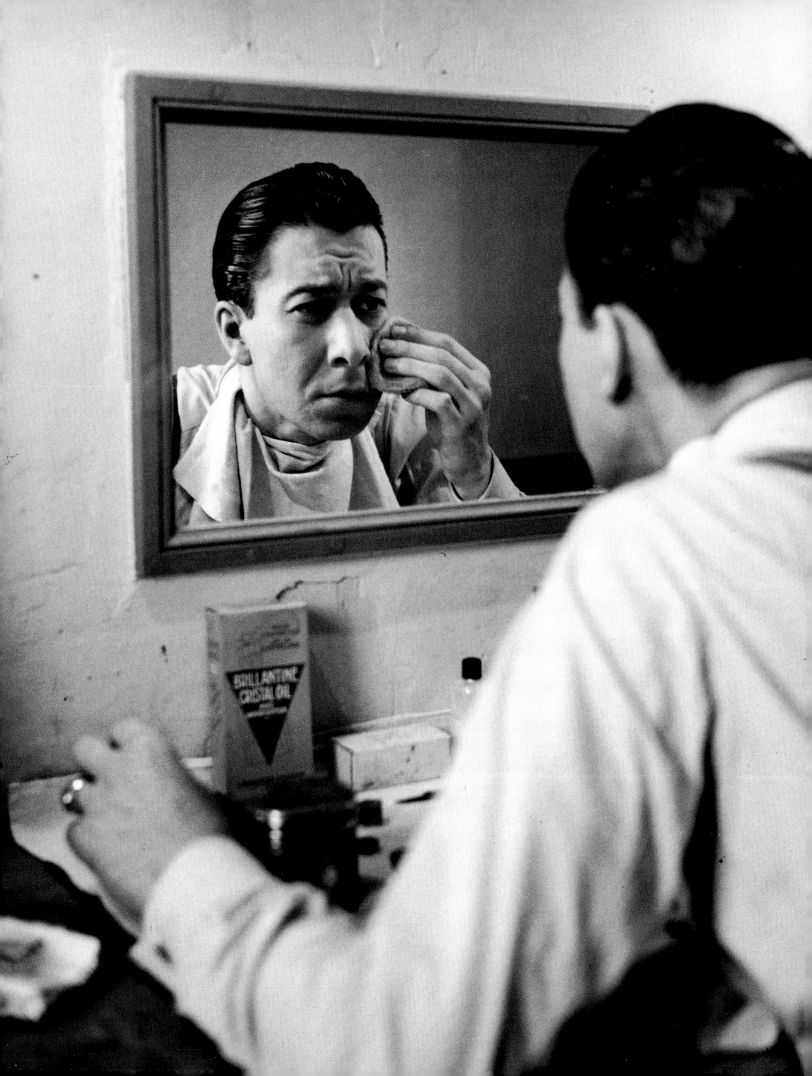

Shrines, alcoves and the stage

Make-up will always be somewhere between nature and culture. On the one hand, visible make-up is used for its intrinsic beauty; this is the cultural aspect. "We had to battle nature, cruel, stupid, wild nature, which we try to outsmart by using every possible ruse of the human spirit," wrote Princess Bibesco, discussing the first beauty parlors in the 1920s. On the other hand make-up is used as an expression in and of itself, used merely to glorify what already exists, what is here: "The ultimate in artifice is to appear natural," wrote Paul Poiret during this same Belle Époque, "but what a sublime nature!"

Skin was most likely the first surface ever painted, long before stone and, of course, canvas. We can assume that early man, participating in magical ceremonial rituals in painted caves, had also painted their bodies.

Make-up followed on from body painting for religious and theatrical purposes. It was used for everything, except for self-expression; it was viewed more like an escape, a mask. A face painted with conventional forms demonstrates that someone else—a god or famous figure—inhabited the actor or the priest. The officiant or the actor had the god or figure inside him and on his skin; the medium was no longer a thin

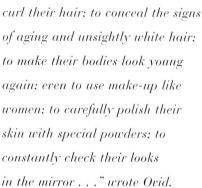

"The men of this century also take care of their appearance. Spouses will follow the fashion of women. . . . They like to be shaved, to have their whiskers taken off; to carefully curl their hair; to conceal the signs of aging and unsightly white hair; to make their bodies look young again; even to use make-up like women; to carefully polish their skin with special powders; to constantly check their looks in the mirror . . ." wrote Ovid.

Robespierre always appeared freshly powdered, and Napoleon abandoned this fashion only after his Italian campaign. He soon became an enthusiastic adept of eau de Cologne, which he used immoderately.

General de Gaulle himself— seemingly so unconcerned by questions of appearance—had himself made up for each of his televised speeches and for his most important press conferences. From 1962 to 1969, he used the services of a film professional, Charly Koubesserian, perhaps because this was the same person used by Brigitte Bardot, who was Marianne on the French stamps—in other words, a symbol of France itself.

Not for women only . . .

Painted from life

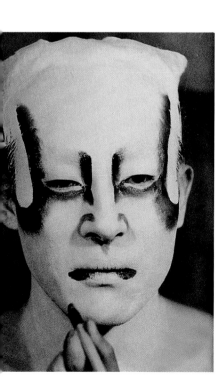

Kabuki actor Minosuke Bando (another Bando is often depicted in prints by Kunisada). The *kumadori* make-up, based on that used in Chinese opera, was introduced to kabuki theater by the actor Danjuro (1660–1704). Top: The eye of the master: Mr. Shu Uemura, founder of the product line of the same name. Far left: Paul Meurisse in the early years of his double career in theater (here in Angers) and in film, July 1941.

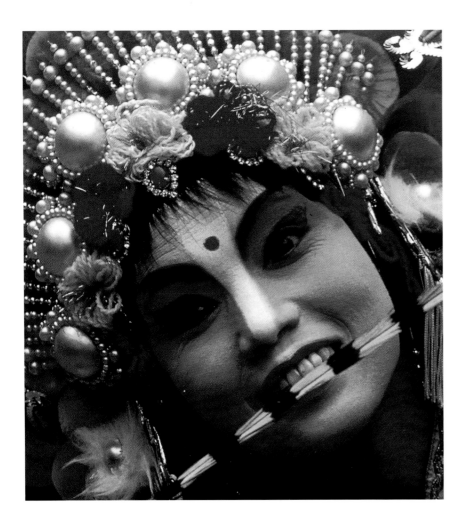

Pink China from the
Sichuan provincial opera
between the Blue River
and the Red Basin.
Right: *Luna,* the serenity
and silent cries of *buto*
dancers, 1986.

invisible film: through the other, he was inhabited and clothed.

On closer examination, what differentiates the "outrageous" make-up of a courtesan from that of an "honest" woman is not necessarily excess; it is rather that the first perpetuates the idea of ceremonial make-up. Throughout history, courtesans were seen more as shrines. In Corinth, for example, more than one thousand courtesans, known as *hierodules*, lived in the complex around Aphrodite's Temple. And the dancing girls of India, known as bayaderes, "essential ornaments for the gods and for private festivities," who resided within the sacred walls, were *devadasis*—servants to the gods.

Even the lowliest prostitute knows a man is not looking specifically for her—Yolande or Amanda—but seeks another through her, the eternal Woman or the figure known only to the unconscious. Her make-up is not overdone; it is symbolic: it is the archetype of femininity depicted with thick strokes of green, red and black. Make-up needs only to sketch "woman" across a face, and this name becomes clearly visible via the gaudy elements that are the mouth, cheekbones and eyes.

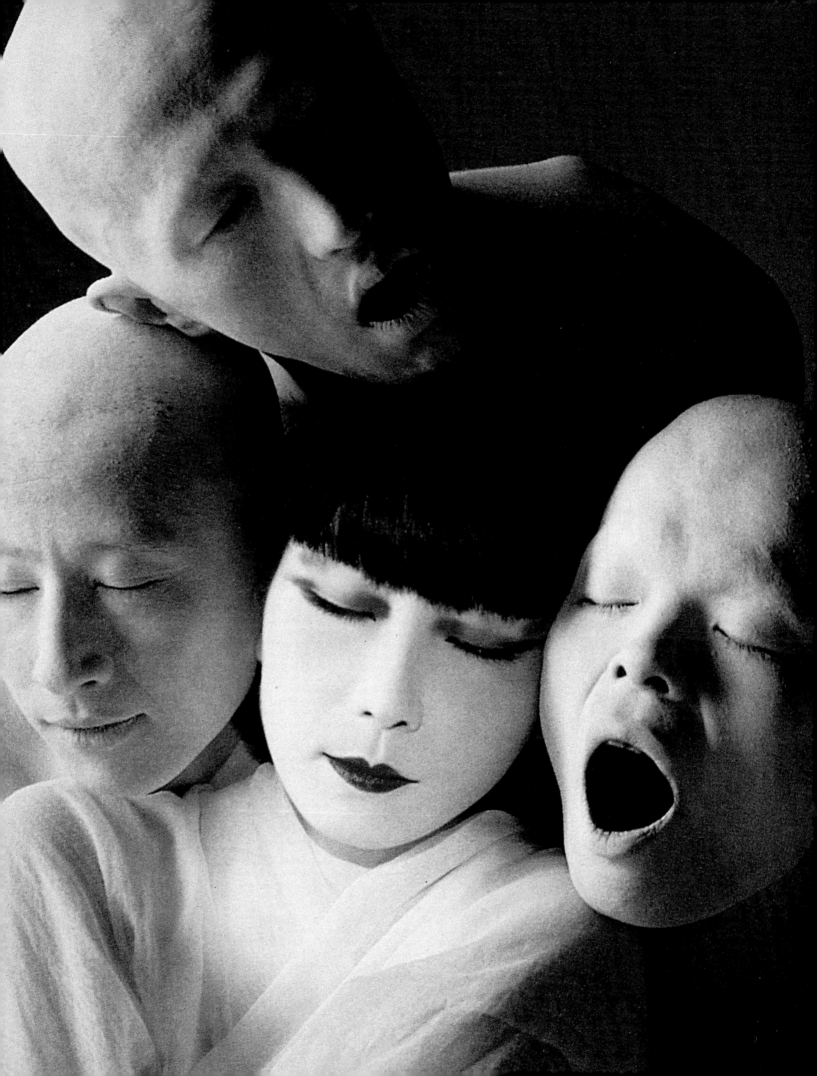

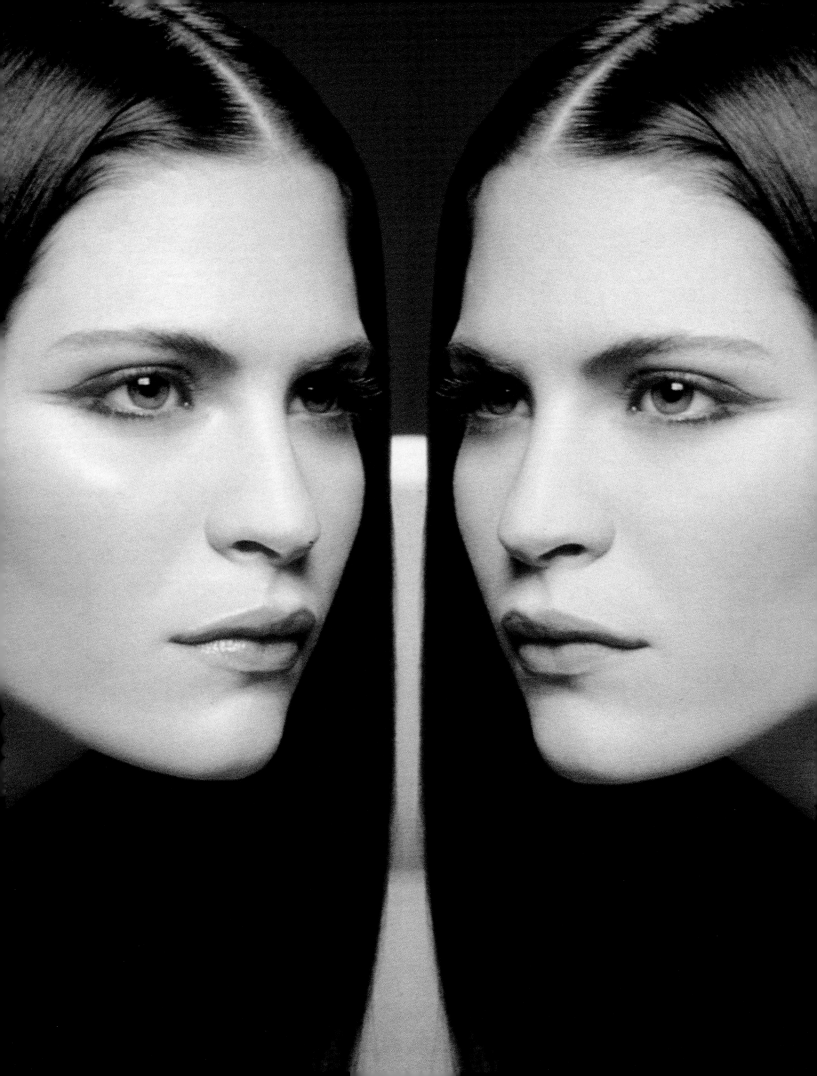

Reality and appearance

This duality of nature and culture, of self-expression and ritual adopted a third form: that of beauty care and treatment as opposed to make-up. The Greeks distinguished between cosmetics and *commoticus*. The first term designated the art of adornment, including everything that enhanced natural beauty (jewels and ornamental accessories) as well as products for protecting and maintaining this natural beauty (beauty care and hygiene products). The second term encompassed the art of disguise, in other words, covering up what was natural or even faulty—or at least that which was merely mediocre. This was the technique for courtesans and the lazy; make-up required less effort than upkeep, said Plato, more or less, in *Giorgias:* in other words, obtaining a relatively inexpensive beauty mask meant that you could avoid an effort that would, however, provide more long-lasting and true effects.

Therefore, our use of the word "cosmetics" today is not entirely correct; we should reserve it for beauty care; *commoticus* should be the proper term for make-up. According to Galen, cosmetics are medicinal, while make-up is harmful. From this point of view, and even leaving aside massages and other

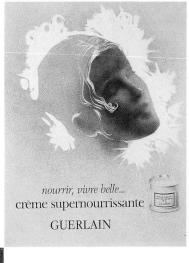

Advertising for beauty treatment and powders by two major brands: Guerlain and Caron, 1950s.

nourrir, vivre belle...
crème supernourrissante
GUERLAIN

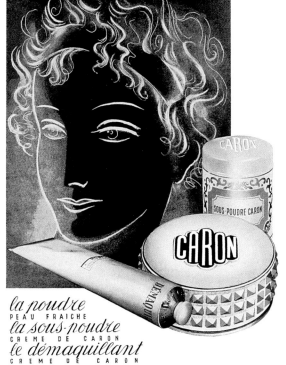

la poudre
PEAU FRAICHE
la sous-poudre
CREME DE CARON
le démaquillant
CREME DE CARON

Far left: Twin set by Guerlain. Make-up today aims to reinforce a woman's identity rather than to modify it.

Painted from life

therapeutic methods, beauty care products penetrate and act from within. Make-up, however, acts on the surface, creates appearances. Cosmetics versus *commoticus* reflects the opposition between depth and surface, even between reality and appearance—although this distinction is less straightforward today than in earlier eras. There is not a single make-up product that doesn't claim to nourish, tighten, or at least moisturize as it covers. These characteristics are presented as curative. Even if we examine the covering aspect alone, the contemporary viewpoint about make-up is far more about internal aspects, as an expression of one's personality. Make-up no longer masks and conceals; it reveals.

We could probably associate make-up trends with the specific self-image of any particular era. In a Balzac novel, the characters—the fictional ones as well as those from which they were certainly inspired—have so much depth, and are so sure of themselves and their existences that they use no make-up. With the *nouveau roman* and structuralism, the death of the subject and the dissolution of the character, everything that could lead to a concept in which "I am only what I reveal" announces the return of visible make-up.

And the woman becomes public

Make-up has become a phenomenon of the masses as urban centers have grown and women have entered the work force in increasing numbers; indeed, make-up has perhaps become a tool of the trade. No text so bluntly expresses the fact that the working woman is a prostitute, whose employee is therefore her pimp, than the following preface to a directory for the cosmetics industry by Paul Guth. Yet his argument in favor of make-up is anything but a denunciation or a cry of indignation. And it was written in 1968!

"For the working woman, beauty has become the leading guarantee of efficiency. Pretty women, such as secretaries, salesgirls in department stores and receptionists of all kinds attract more customers than the others. In earlier days, only a husband or lover had rights to a woman's beauty. Today, the public has replaced these two privileged beings. The actress is beautiful for an entire audience. A working woman has become an actress. She is beautiful for everyone. Her beauty is an asset for the company that hired her. A woman's beauty is an essential element of the daily performance that the century has put on for itself in the working world."

Relegated to the status of a marketable good, recorded on the

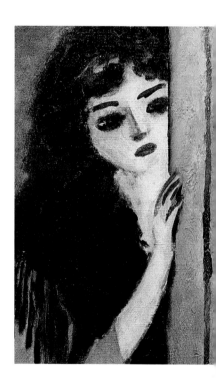

Conceal or reveal? *The Gypsy* (or *The Curious One*) by van Dongen, 1910–1911. Right: The fatal beauty of Maria Felix, Yves Montand's friend in *Les Héros sont fatigués* by Yves Ciampi, 1955.

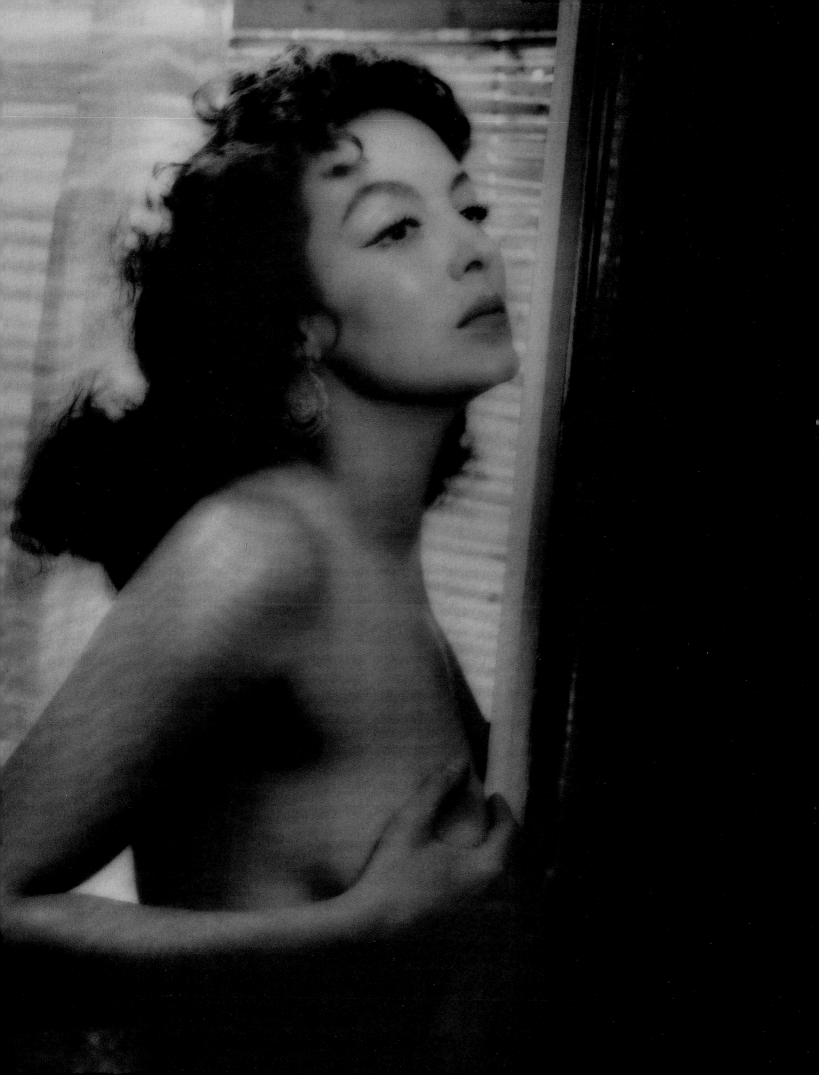

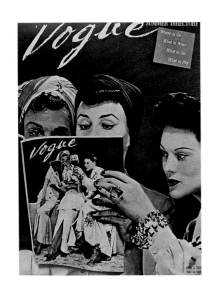

The Atlantic route was
cut off by the war,
so America sought to
create its own fashions:
Vogue, 1941.
Right: Postwar beauty.

accounting sheets, considered the personal property of a company, women would, on the contrary—after the hippie trends of post-1968—adopt a cosmetic fashion that stressed identity, that emphasized individualism and self-expression.

Before becoming a "public woman," the housewife already had the prostitute, courtesan and actress as role models. If she wanted to be more than an "extra" in her own house, if she wanted a role of her own, she had to seduce her husband, catch his eye and therefore compete with the public woman—but on her own private stage. Everyone knows that you get someone's attention first through your looks, then by your inheritance; it's no coincidence that courtesans have almost always been, and continue to be, blond, because blond—white to be more exact—is the most visible color, as it reflects 84 percent of the light that strikes it.

Seduction begins at home. This was especially true for an ancient Greek woman; she rarely left home, but if she did, it was unthinkable to wear make-up. With the exception of the Dionysian festivals, during which the revelers slathered their faces with chalk, make-up was banned for women.

"Only courtesans, who were often of Oriental origin, used beauty products on a regular basis," wrote Pinset. In Greece in the fourth century B.C., as make-up was considered to be part of a courtesan's accoutrements, the word always had a pejorative meaning in texts. In Rome, the fashionable perfumer Cosmus, mentioned by Martial, had one scent known as *jonc odorant,* which was reserved for courtesans.

In the third century A.D., Tertullian wrote indignantly: "What is more scandalous than to see Christian women, the inviolable guardians of purity, as adorned and embellished as courtesans? What difference is there then between you and these unfortunate victims of impurity? In early days, strict laws separated them from matrons and did not allow them to wear the adornments of higher-class people; we can see the licentiousness of this century, which grows more insolent every day, putting these miserable creatures on an equal plane with famous ladies—without being able to distinguish one from the other. Thus the Holy Scriptures tell us face make-up and adornments are the marks of a prostituted body."

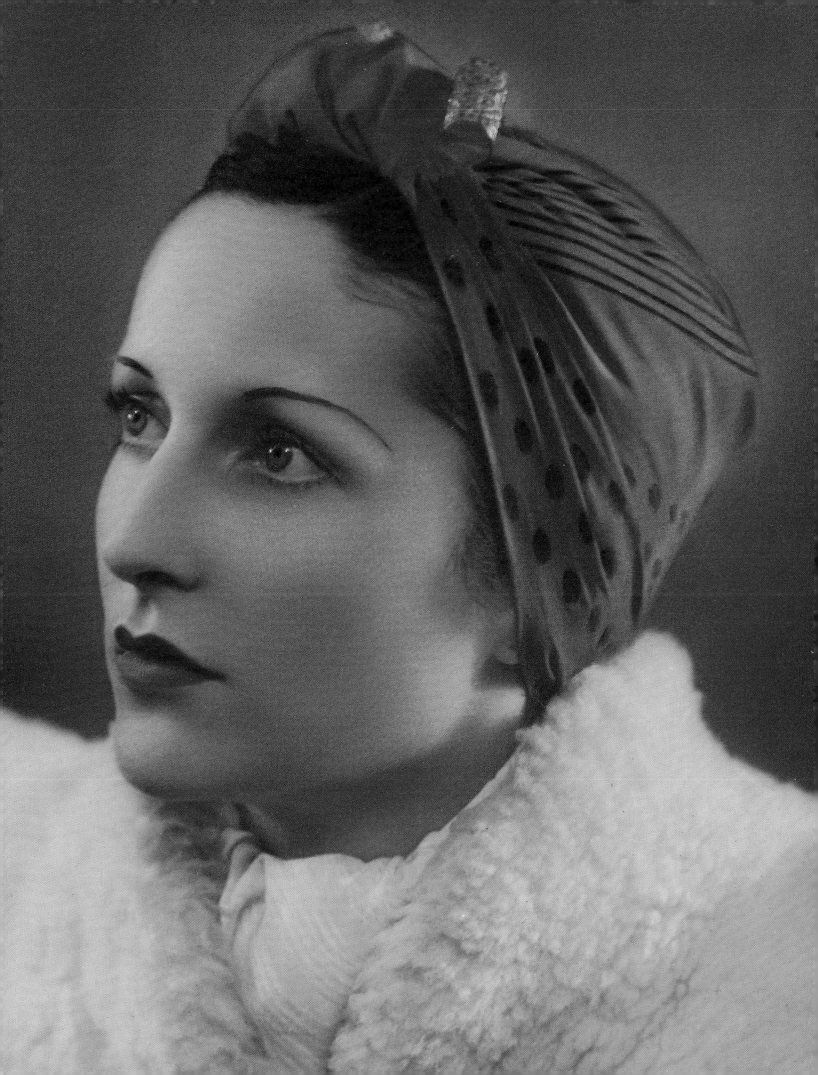

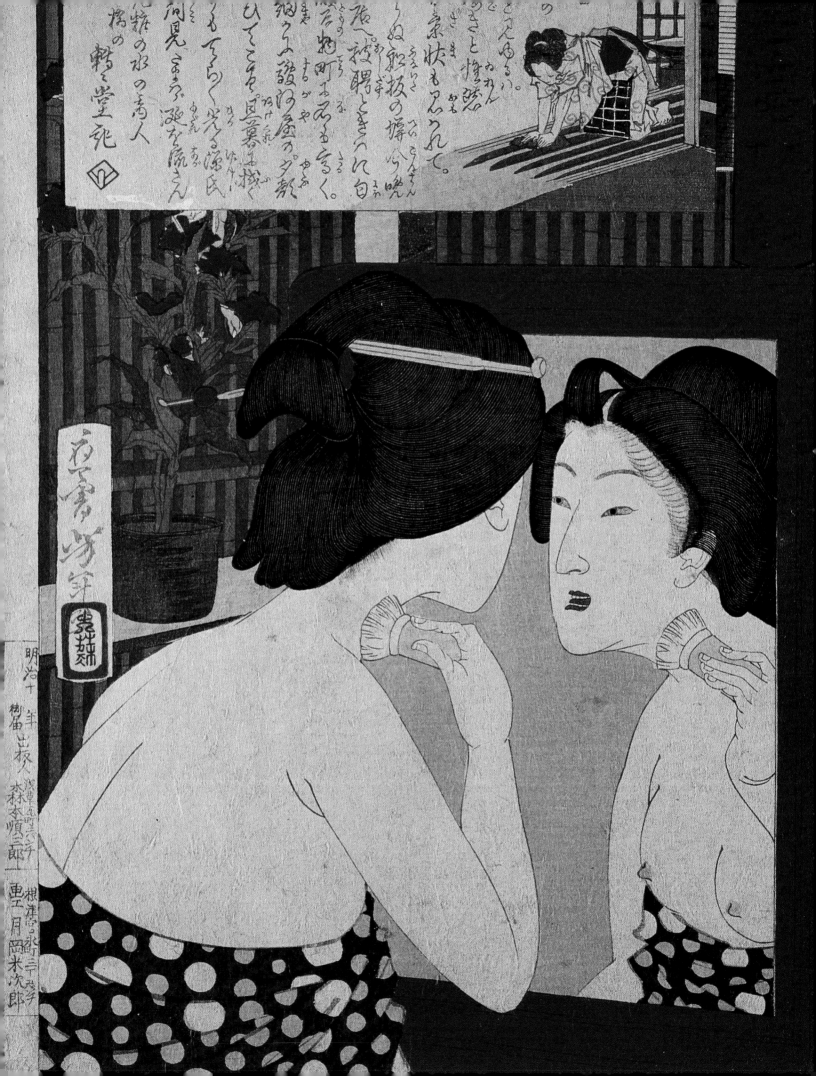

Everybody on stage

It became clear that women had to battle their dangerous rivals, the courtesans, on their own terms; the task was made easier by the courtesans themselves, who were free with their advice and generously made their cosmetic skills available to everyone. Aspasia, for whom Pericles repudiated his wife, published a series of precepts for maintaining health and beauty from 375 to 370. Many of these, according to René Cerbelaud, were recopied by Criton. Galen cited the book that Cleopatra—the queen who had several Roman kings at her feet—wrote concerning beauty products, as well as another that the Greek poetess Elephantis wrote for courtesans in the late first century B.C.

In the second half of the relatively unembellished nineteenth century, Lola Montès published her *Art de la Beauté, ou Secrets de la toilette des dames* (The Art of Beauty, or Secrets of a Woman's Toilette). Note that she, even more than her fellow courtesans, was democratic—she not only shared her secrets, she was also the reason for the abdication of the king of Bavaria. Indeed, inspired by this event, a satirist wrote that "all women of questionable virtue are, at this time, concerned with liberal constitutions;

The time factor

The courtesans of Yoshiwara got up around noon, took a bath, ate breakfast, then took various artistic lessons. They then started to put on their make-up at 2 p.m., spending an amount of time that can be calculated according to the number of combs and tortoiseshell pins they used in the hair—a figure that grew larger as the century progressed, exceeding twenty on a print by Kunisada in 1825. Granted, this is not entirely specific information, but as regards the First Empire in France, quasi-scientific data exists: Empress Marie-Louise received the gift of a dressing table, which includes a music box that could play for 45 minutes. As we can assume that the music was designed to keep the empress entertained for the entire time she was working on her make-up, this would seem to be a fairly reliable indication of the time it took her imperial highness (and archduchess of Austria) to get ready in the early 1810s. One hundred and fifty years later, Helena Rubenstein, working in her New York beauty institute, developed "a make-up technique that would take no more than fifteen minutes and would not require any touchups throughout the day." The application of the eyeliner, which only involved the upper eyelids, took the longest time of all, four minutes; lips and eyebrows could be made up in just two minutes.

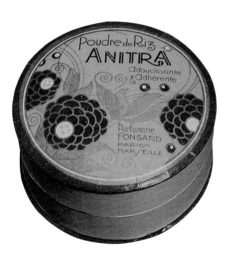

Rice powder (starch).
Left: The *ukiyo-e* genre —scenes of everyday life— only appeared with the development of the print in the second half of the seventeenth century. Colored prints appeared one century later. These prints depicted mostly actors and courtesans. *Woman with a Brush,* Meiji period, 1868–1912.

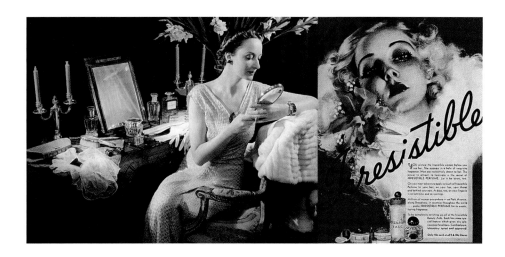

Between two mirrors, as
illustrated by *Harper's Bazaar*
in 1936, and Irresistible
Cosmetics lipstick in 1937.
Right: Michèle Morgan.
As French actor Jean Gabin
could have said, "You have
beautiful eyes, you know,
even when they're closed!"

they write charters and create
systems. Their noble aim is to
convert all the absolute monarchs by
next spring. The people have hope,
the people are right."

The French word for make-up,
maquillage, comes straight from the
theater, as indicated in Littré's French
dictionary of 1877: "This is no longer
a theater term; many women now
make themselves up." The practice
of making oneself up comes from the
theater, but a far more ancient one. In
the eastern cities of the Late
Byzantine Empire, theater had
become high society's favorite
pastime, and the actress, the new
female role model. Furthermore, as
women went out more often, other
social areas became places where
they could show off—with the church
one of the leading venues. Here we
see the Temple of Reality has
become the Temple of Appearance;
and the basilica, its theater.

The church obviously viewed this
cosmetic display as a lack of respect
toward divine creation, which surely
had no need of improvement, and
the church fathers unanimously
condemned the actors and the
faithful audiences.

"What so grievously offends [our
Lord] is the extravagant attention
with which several women use one
hundred kinds of ingredients to
make their skin white and uniform,
to make up their faces, to color their
cheeks with vermilion, to blacken
their eyes with soot. God's work
undoubtedly displeases them; they
find fault with it; they condemn the
wisdom of the sovereign creator of
all things," wrote Tertullian. He
continued in his *Treaty against
Performances*: "Do you also believe
that God cherishes the actor, who so
carefully shaves his beard, thereby
disfiguring through this infidelity the
face that has been given to him?"

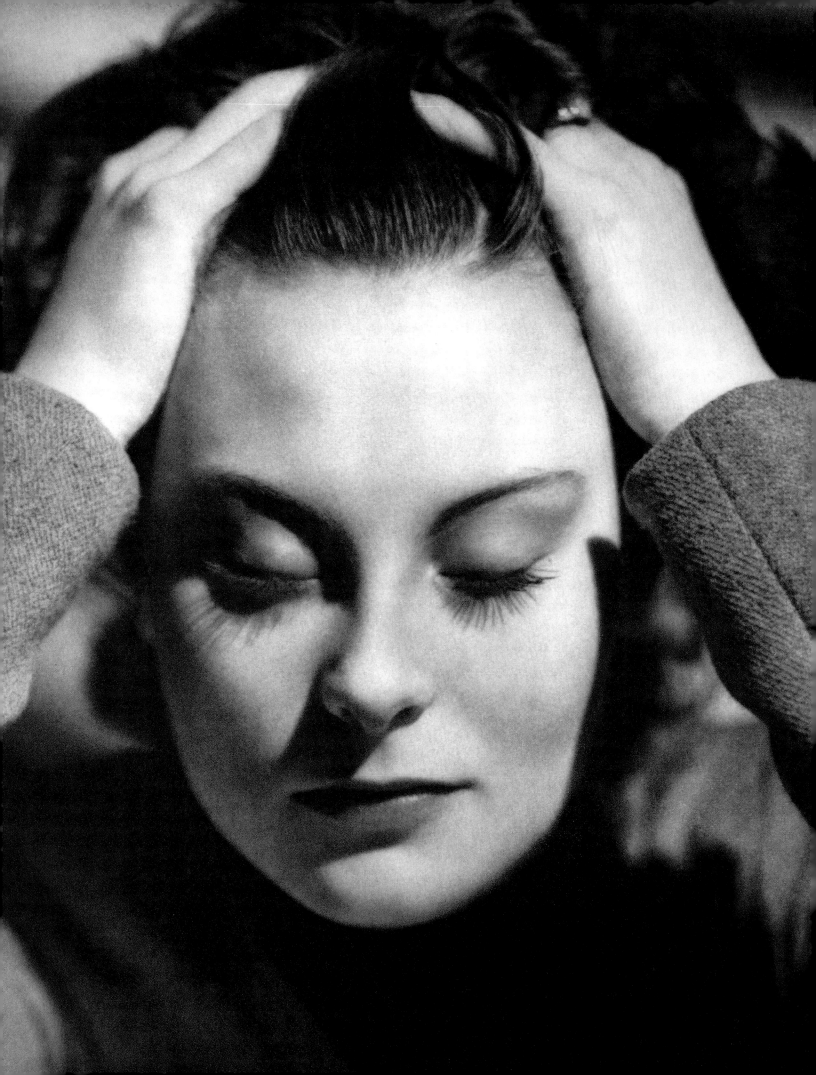

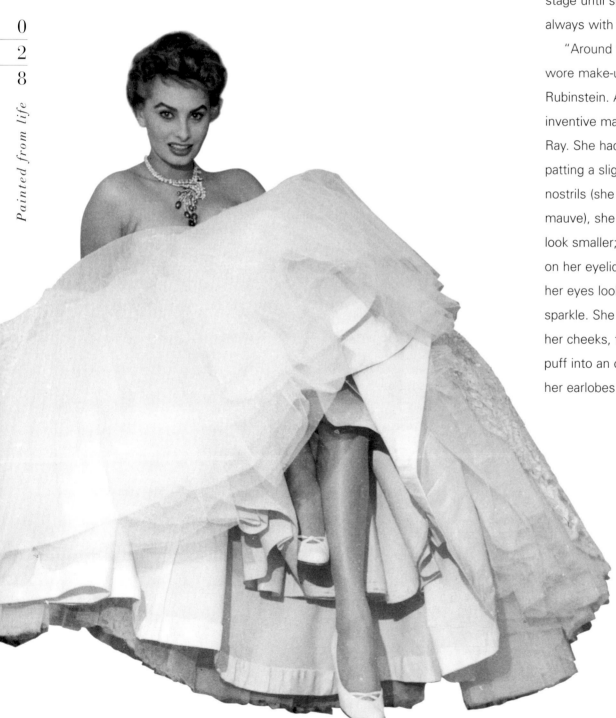

Sophia Loren. First noticed
during a beauty pageant,
she would star in
The Millionairess, in 1960,
by Anthony Asquith.

Painted from life

How to marry a millionaire

In the mid-nineteenth century,
courtesans and actresses remained
the last women to maintain a gaudy
style of make-up. Mlle Mars was
sometimes mocked for the
aggressive make-up she wore until
the last night of her life; this
anecdote was repeated often, yet
she continued to play ingénues on
stage until she was sixty—and
always with tremendous success.

"Around 1908, only actresses
wore make-up," wrote Helena
Rubinstein. Among them, the most
inventive may have been Gabrielle
Ray. She had discovered that by
patting a slight bit of make-up on her
nostrils (she used spots of red and
mauve), she could make her nose
look smaller; using a little make-up
on her eyelids and temples made
her eyes look larger and added a
sparkle. She also blended rouge on
her cheeks, then dipped a powder
puff into an ocher powder to color
her earlobes and the tip of her chin."

Just before World War I broke out, fashionable artists created and signed artwork used in cosmetics advertisements, thereby giving a sign of approval to the use of these products. The budding movie industry created a star system and with it, a desire to emulate these lovely creatures. "Hollywood is the source of the modern cosmetics industry. Beauty treatment provided to stars by Max Factor and Elizabeth Arden, and the unguents and make-up created for them have spread to every face around the world," noted Edgar Morin.

Yet on closer examination, the message is more subtle. When Lauren Bacall appeared in a soap advertisement—"If nine out of ten movie stars use the Lux Beauty Bar..."—the caption under her photograph and her name reads: "Star of Cinemascope film in Technicolor: *How to Marry a Millionaire*." The concept is not to offer the customer the beauty of an admired actress; it is to send the message that, if she uses the same beauty products, she could be like the actress—who managed to marry a millionaire on screen—but could also put these assets to use for the same goal in real life.

Cosmetics have remained the front-line weapon in any marriage strategy. As early as 1770, the English parliament decreed that "any woman of any age of any condition, virgin, daughter or widow, who deceived and drew into marriage one of Her Majesty's subject through the use of perfume, fake hair . . . high-heeled shoes or any other unfair maneuvers, shall be subject to the punishments associated with sorcery, and the marriage shall be annuled." Henry VIII repudiated Anne of Cleves, claiming that he had been deceived by an overly flattering portrait painted by Holbein—an argument that could be considered convincing, as oil paint can alter surfaces much as make-up does.

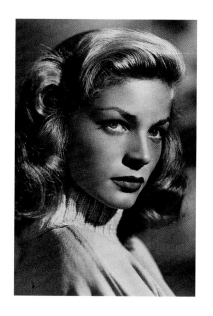

Lauren Bacall in 1946, just after her marriage to Humphrey Bogart. She filmed *How to Marry a Millionaire* in 1953.

Painted from life

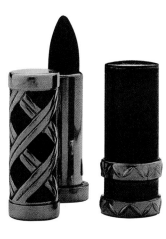

Versailles case by Lancôme, made of lacquer and criss-crossed with a gold motif.

Chanel, in *Vogue USA,*
summer of 1942.
Right: Solange David by
J.-H. Lartigue, 1929.
In this case, the lipstick
creates a vertical swath.

A colorful geography

"A woman's toilette is the array of all the powders, all the essences, all the make-up intended to alter a person, and to transform age and even ugliness into youth and beauty. This is where all the lines are corrected, where eyebrows are reshaped, where teeth are replaced, where a face is created; where, finally, a woman changes her form and her skin. This is where the delectable *Siphonia* gathers together her suitors, newswriters, dogs and abbots; and where the precious *Dorillas* receives new brochures, reads the preface and the titles, and learns what the Comedy is all about," according to Caraccioli's dictionary.

The ceremony is the same on each and every continent. Edmond de Goncourt, in *Outamaro,* describes the scene as it is depicted in Japanese prints: "A metal mirror placed on a lacquered stand, covered with a piece of embroidered silk; rice powder for the face, rice powder for the neck, make-up for the lips, black for the teeth. . ."

When Sonnini traveled to Egypt, he noted that "nowhere are women so uniformly beautiful; nowhere do they more skillfully master the talent of assisting nature; nowhere, in other words, are they more clever or experienced in the art of stopping the passage of time, an art that is based on a wide diversity of practical recipes."

This is the result of thousands of years of experience. If he could have traveled through time to Pharaonic Egypt, Sonnini would have been able to see a land so enamored of cosmetics that people were sometimes their own perfume-braziers, their own incense-burners: during celebrations, men, women, children and servants could all wear the famous cone of fat, often called a Theban cone, placed atop their hair—whether real or a wig. Like a cake of sugar molded with scented oils and probably stuck with seeds of myrrh, this cone was designed to melt slowly during receptions and banquets, first dripping down the face, then down the arms. It was often replaced with a new cone and frequently adorned with a lotus flower.

La Celestina, one of the three principal characters in Spanish literature along with Don Quixote and Don Juan, is both made up and a make-up artist: "An old whore whose eyes are lined with kohl; a perfumer and master in the art of concocting make-up. She prepared purified mixtures, cooked up make-up, polish, glossy tinctures and lightening lotions for the skin. And still other lotions for the face: grated asphodel, bladder-nut tree, serpentaria, earth-gall, verjuice, all distilled and sweetened. . . . To

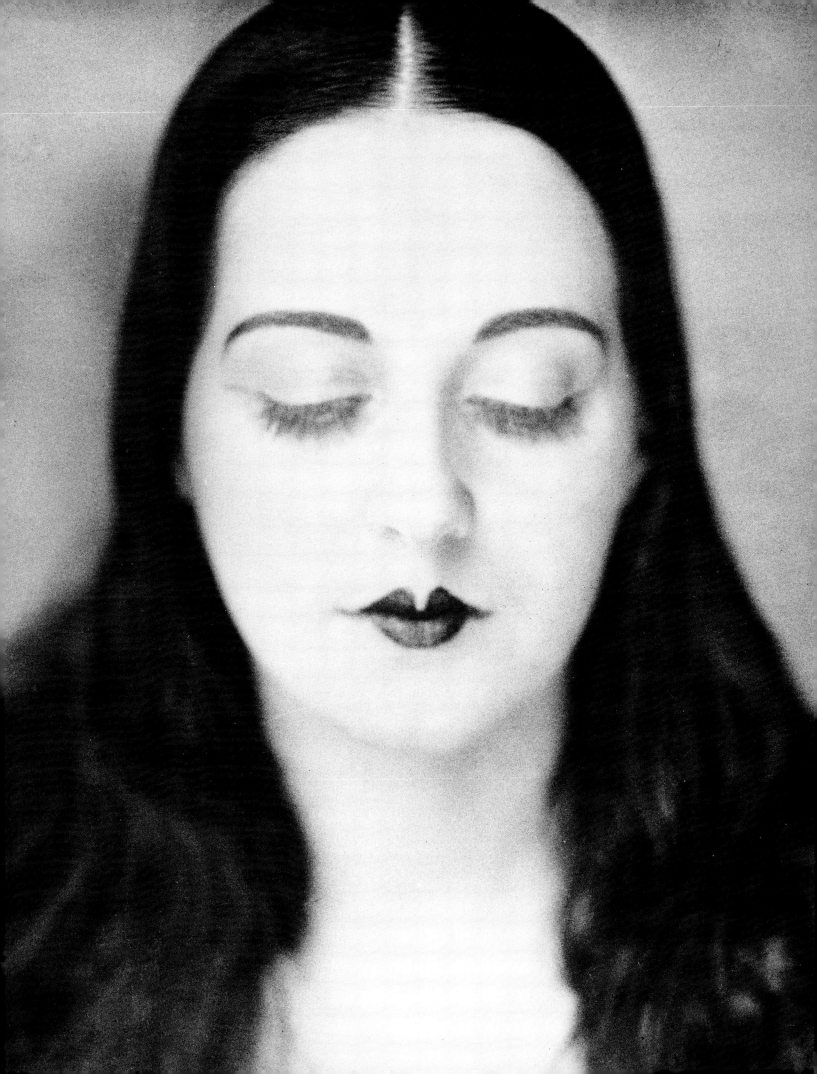

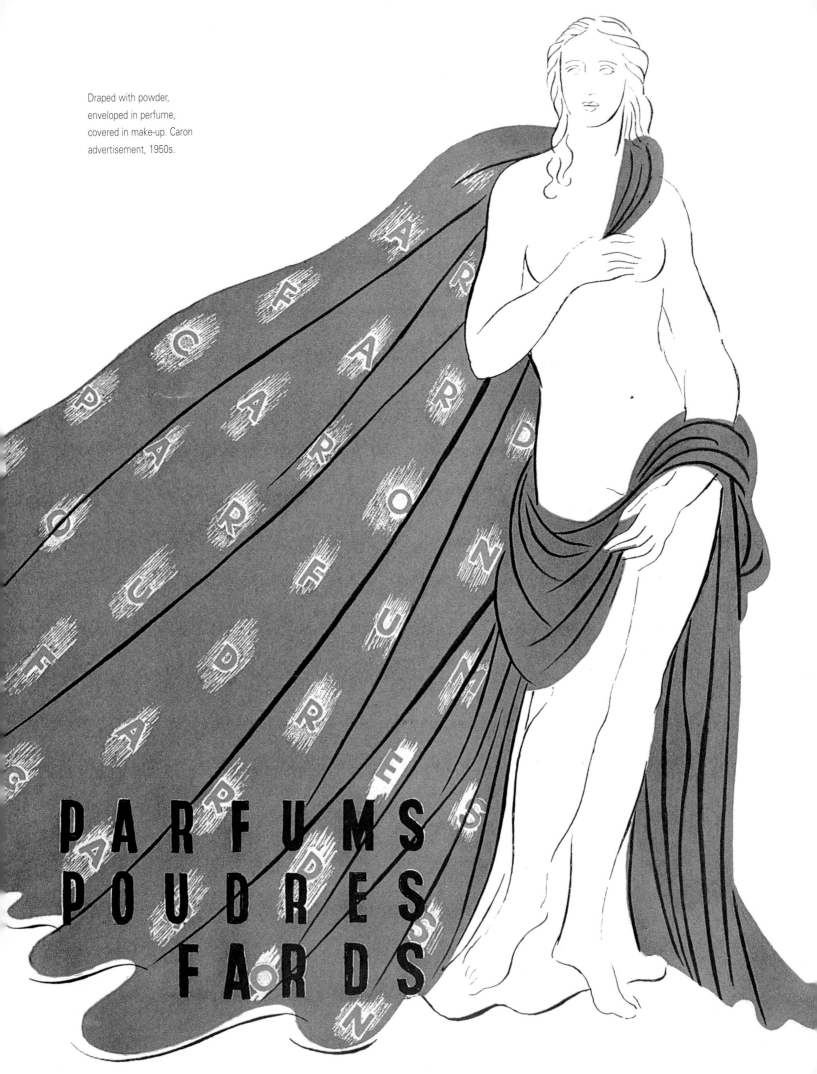

Draped with powder,
enveloped in perfume,
covered in make-up. Caron
advertisement, 1950s.

lighten skin, she prepared concoctions of vine shoots, holm oak, rye and marrubium, with saltpeter, alum, millefeuille and still other ingredients. . . . What diverse oils she prepared for the face! It's unbelievable! Storax, jasmine, alluvium, fruit pips, violets, tincture of benzoin, pistachio, pinion, small seeds, jujube, corn-cockle, lupin, vetch, hazelnut and birdseed."

Kalidasa, one of the greatest poets of India, who lived from about A.D. 390 to 460 described beautiful women "drawing lines of make-up on their flower faces, filling their hair with aloe smoke. . . . Fragrant liana, scented wood, saffron; these beautiful women, languishing from desire, apply make-up to their breasts, also using sandalwood

mixed with musk." He continued: "Joyful, beautiful from the make-up on their lips, their breath sweetened by betel nut . . ." In his writings, even nature uses make-up, and he depicts the seasons by comparing them to make-up. During the rainy season, for example: "Clouds dark as the petals of blue water lilies fill the sky from all directions, looking like crushed antimony."

Cosmetics were produced in every land bordering the Mediterranean Sea, particularly the two largest cities in the empire, after Rome: Alexandria in Egypt, and Antioch in Asia Minor; in Corinth, Greece and in Capua, Italy. In this city an entire street, Seplasia, was occupied by cosmetic-makers; they were known as the Seplasiarii.

Woodbury,
Matched Make-Up, 1930s.

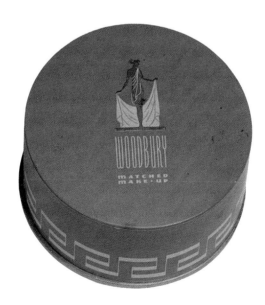

Painted from life

A toiletry case decorated
with ivory caryatids and
containing make-up tools;
Roman era, Cumae,
first-third centuries.

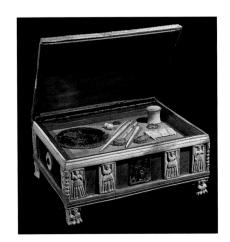

As Above, As Below

On Olympus, the gods themselves, including Zeus's spouse Hera, first among equals and who could be considered perfect by nature, all needed beauty products: "First of all, ambrosia eliminates from her desirable body all blemishes. She then anoints herself with a thick, divine and smooth oil, whose scent is made specially for her. When she sprinkles it in Zeus's palaces on the bronze doorway, the scent fills the air and the earth. She anoints her beautiful body with it, then combs her hair with her own hands, and braids them into glistening tresses, which hang, beautiful and divine, from her eternal forehead."

In the Bible, which we can situate somewhere between heaven and earth, when Jezebel, Athaliah's mother, learns that Jehu has arrived from Samaria, she paints her eyes before appearing before the usurper, in an effort to calm his anger. Judith, before going to meet Holofernes, probably paid more attention to her dress than her make-up per se, but in any case, once she had stepped out of her widow's dress, paid a great deal of attention to her appearance and to her hair, using large quantities of unguents.

Our Painter Who is in Heaven . . . could perhaps be the prayer intoned by Gregory of Nazianzus, when he wrote of the pink cheeks of the modest: "This is the color given to us by our Painter." On a more down-to-earth level, this principle is sometimes embodied by the professional painter who is called upon to work directly from life: "As a practicing artist, you will sometimes have to shade or paint living flesh, for example, the color of men's and women's faces. For this, you can soften your colors with eggs or, even better, cover it with oil or liquid varnish, which is the strongest tempera that exists." The varnish recommended by Andrea Cenini is made from a base of pine or juniper resin. He then used egg yolks and water boiled with bran as a wash over the painted face.

Beauty products and techniques changed very little in the eight to ten centuries preceding and following the start of the Christian era, and stretching from Attica to Asia Minor.

Right: *Judith at the Gates
of Bethulia* (detail). Freedom
conquered through beauty,
as interpreted by Jules-Claude
Ziegler, one of Ingres's
students.

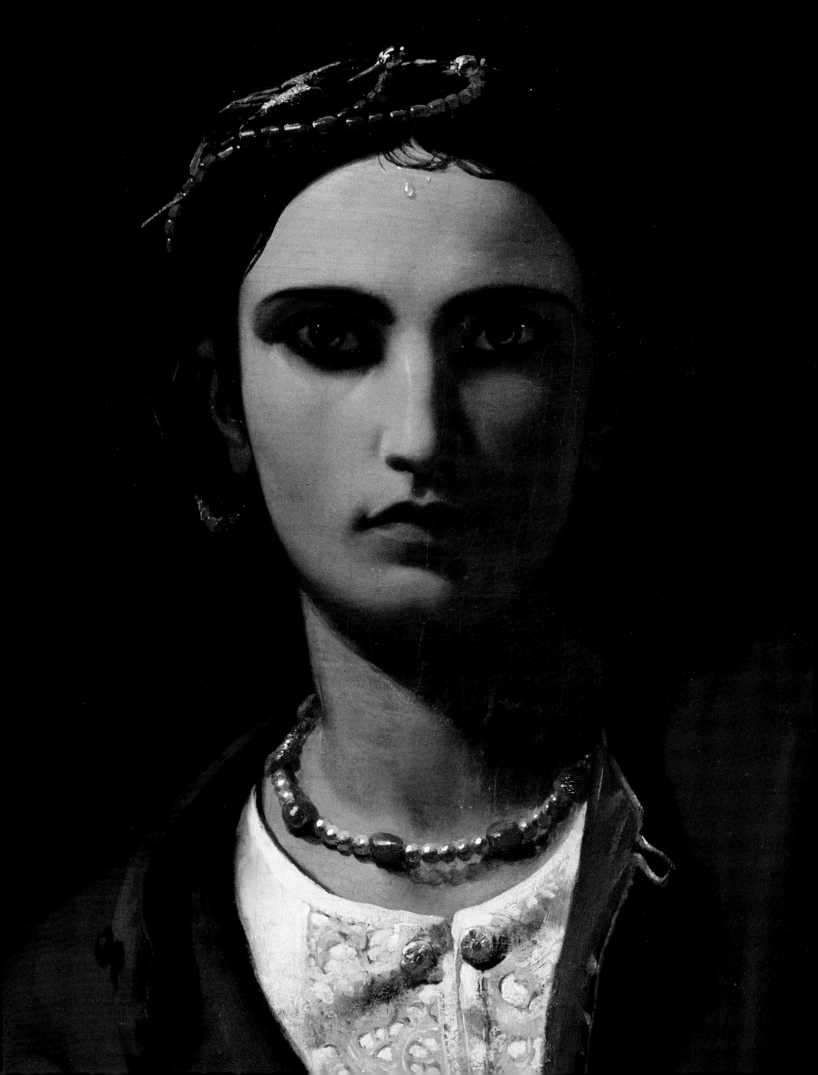

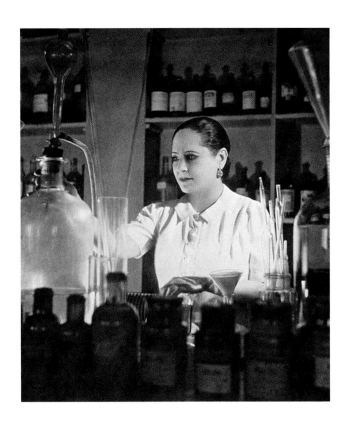

Helena Rubinstein in her laboratory, ca. 1936.
Right: The vamp Theda Bara, for whom she provided make-up—fitting for the actress who would play Cleopatra and, here, Salome, in 1918.

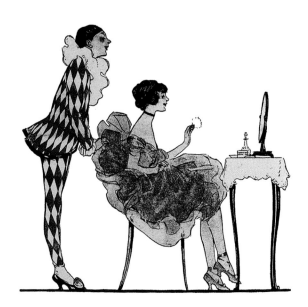

People washed themselves in the Middle Ages and used powder in the Renaissance; the Baroque period tossed out cleanliness and used rouge instead. The nineteenth-century bourgeois rediscovered personal hygiene and scarcely used make-up at all. Our own era arrived without any real change in the situation.

When Helena Rubenstein opened her first French shop, Maisons de Beauté Valaze, in 1912 (four years after London), she wrote: "English women during the years preceding World War I used make-up with extreme discretion, which reduced my field of experience to surface cosmetics, in other words, the artistic creation of a large line of make-up." Parisians, however, "use more make-up and are already thinking of how to create a harmonious balance between their make-up and their attire. The only problem is that the foundation make-up they have is too opaque; with the powder they use, it forms a layer that covers so completely it seems comical today. Yet it was fashion that created this style, by encouraging pale faces often powdered with mauve, or blackened eyes and very red lips."

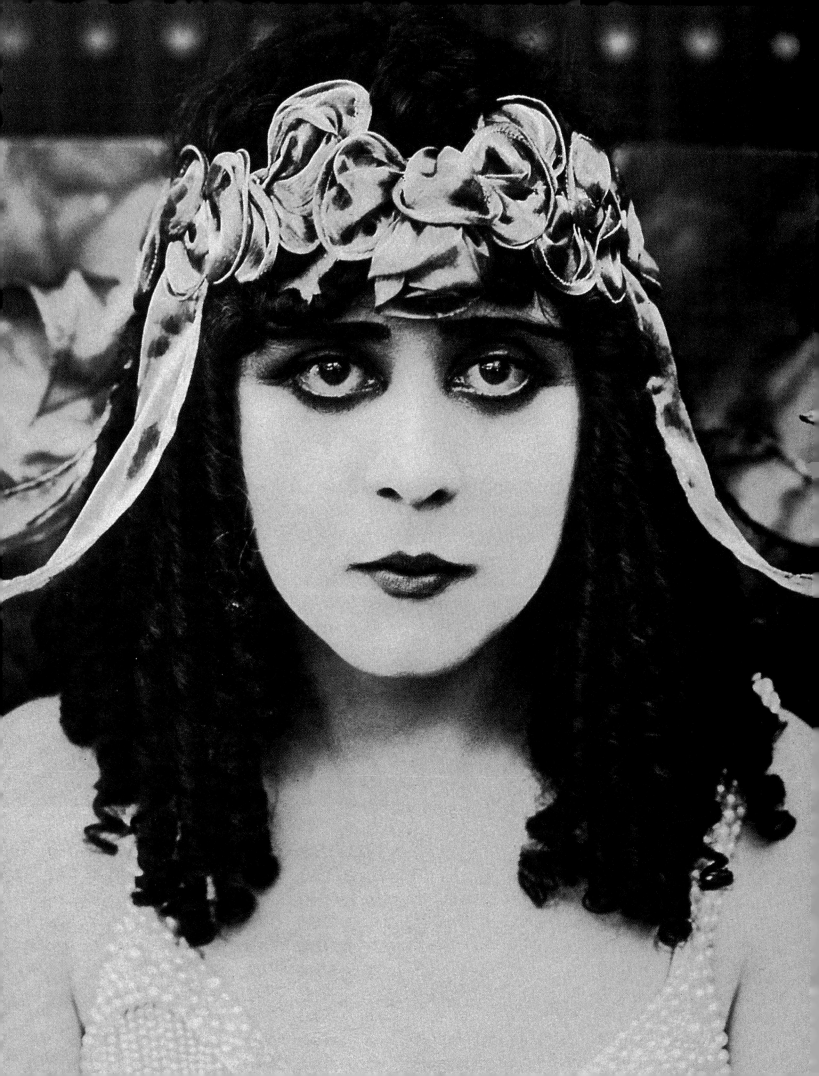

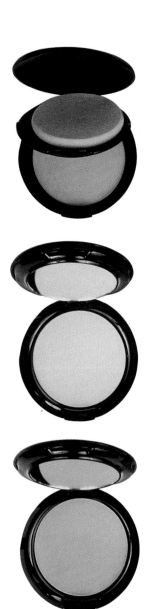

Compact powder on the half-shell, in various shades, by Make Up For Ever. Right: Siegel's "Peach-skin" model, ca. 1925. "At the beginning of each season, a clothed figure called the 'Poupée de France' appeared in Venice on the Merceria; this was the prototype that women were to follow—and any extravagance inspired from this model is beautiful." Goldoni, *Memoirs*, 1787.

Make-up forever

After World War I, Elizabeth Arden, situated at 2 Rue de la Paix in Paris, at the yacht club in Cannes, and in the galleries of the Grand Hotel in Biarritz, offered far more than beauty treatments; her clients came for the luxurious and voluptuous ambience of her salons decorated by Vertès and Drian. Meanwhile, on the street, make-up had become an everyday phenomenon that continued to expand at breakneck speed; even the Stock Market crash of 1929 could not stop it.

"The only American industry that remained unaffected by the widespread economic crisis was the beauty industry. American women continued to spend [in 1930] approximately 70 million dollars per week, 36 billion dollars per year. This was slightly more than double the annual budget of India, if my memory serves me well," wrote Aldous Huxley.

And all of this was done to give them "that hard look" of the machine-woman of *Metropolis*. "In Paris, where this trend was most exaggerated, many women no longer looked human at all. Slathered with oily white and red, they looked like they were wearing masks. You had to look closely to discover the gentle, lively face concealed under this layer.'"

Helena Rubenstein's empire was built around a cream presented to her family by "the famous Polish actress

Modjeska." The statement by Bourjois that it ostensibly "produced products specially for women's beauty" was misleading; at this point, it only produced a single product, essentially designed for actors and actresses. "Color Harmony, a complete line of powders, foundations and lipsticks in shades harmonized for each individual type," was created by Max Factor for all the Hollywood stars—before it then became accessible to every other women dreaming of the screen idols.

Carven was the first fashion house to create beauty products. The owner, Carven, "a prompt and petite Parisian, has a gift for publicity, over and above her talent. Whether she is launching a perfume, a powder, a lipstick or a new dress style, she instantly organizes the perfect party so that all eyes are focused on her creation," extolled the *Guide Odé de Paris* in 1944.

Soon after, Christian Dior created a revolution—of tyranny. "In just a few months, he had forced French women to completely overhaul their wardrobes by lengthening hemlines by some eight inches and getting rid of overstocked fabrics," wrote Georgette Elgey, a historian of the French Fourth Republic. This New Look was accompanied by a perfume, Miss Dior, the one absolutely essential item on any women's dressing table. "How I

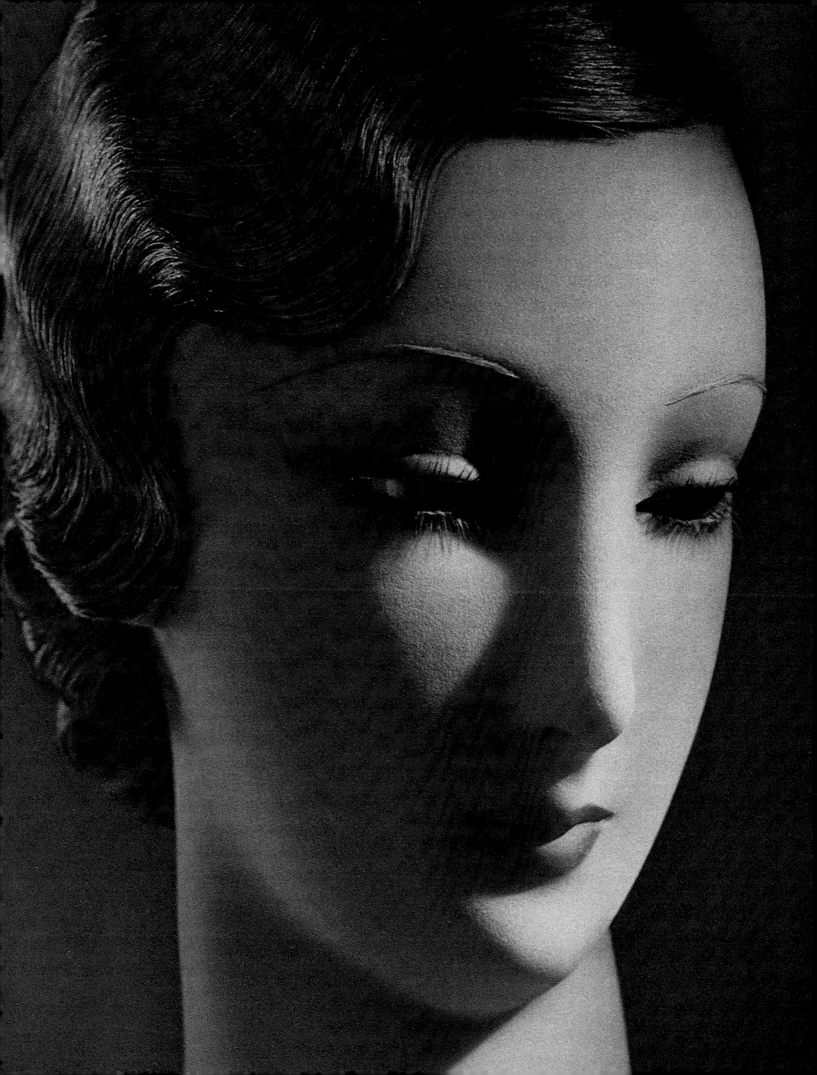

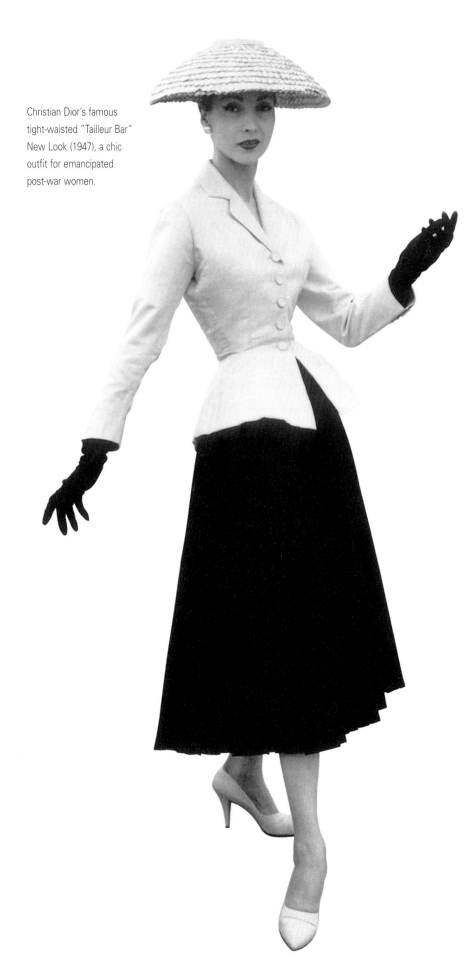

Christian Dior's famous tight-waisted "Tailleur Bar" New Look (1947), a chic outfit for emancipated post-war women.

Painted from life

miss Dior," lamented any Anglo-Saxon woman who had the misfortune of living out of range of a well-stocked luxury perfume store. By this time Christian Dior had become one of the four most famous Frenchmen alive, along with Jean-Paul Sartre, Charles de Gaulle and Pablo Picasso. The fashion designer was extremely well placed for the make-up industry, especially with regard to the prewar concern of French women who were "already thinking of how to create a harmonious balance between their make-up and their attire." On the other hand, a clothes designer creates fashion, which implies codes and standards that apply identically to everyone—something that seems contradictory to today's "fashionable" concept of make-up as self-expression.

Is make-up then a fashion or a statement of individuality? Dior always wanted to create seasonal make-up collections, similar to what was done in clothes design: a spring and autumn look, seasonal interpretations and trends, all in harmony with, or as a counterpoint to, ready-to-wear clothing.

Dior's rouge, 1955, with silver and gold case.

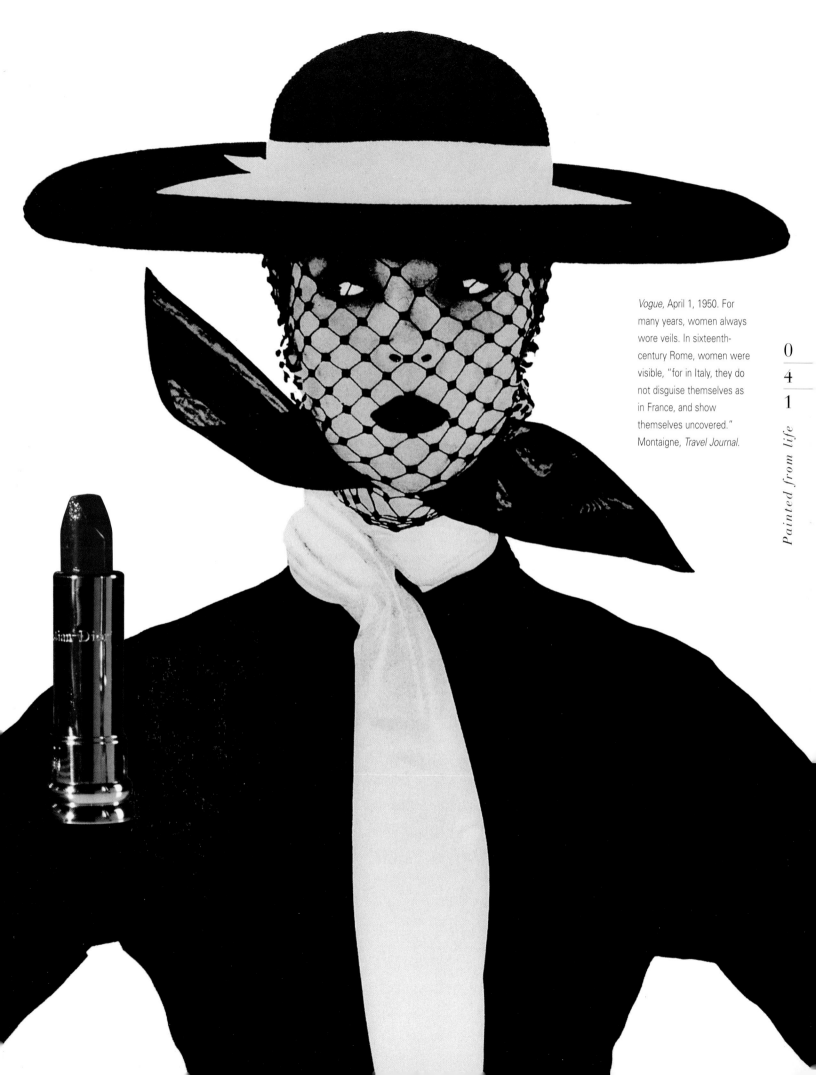

Vogue, April 1, 1950. For many years, women always wore veils. In sixteenth-century Rome, women were visible, "for in Italy, they do not disguise themselves as in France, and show themselves uncovered." Montaigne, *Travel Journal.*

Painted from life

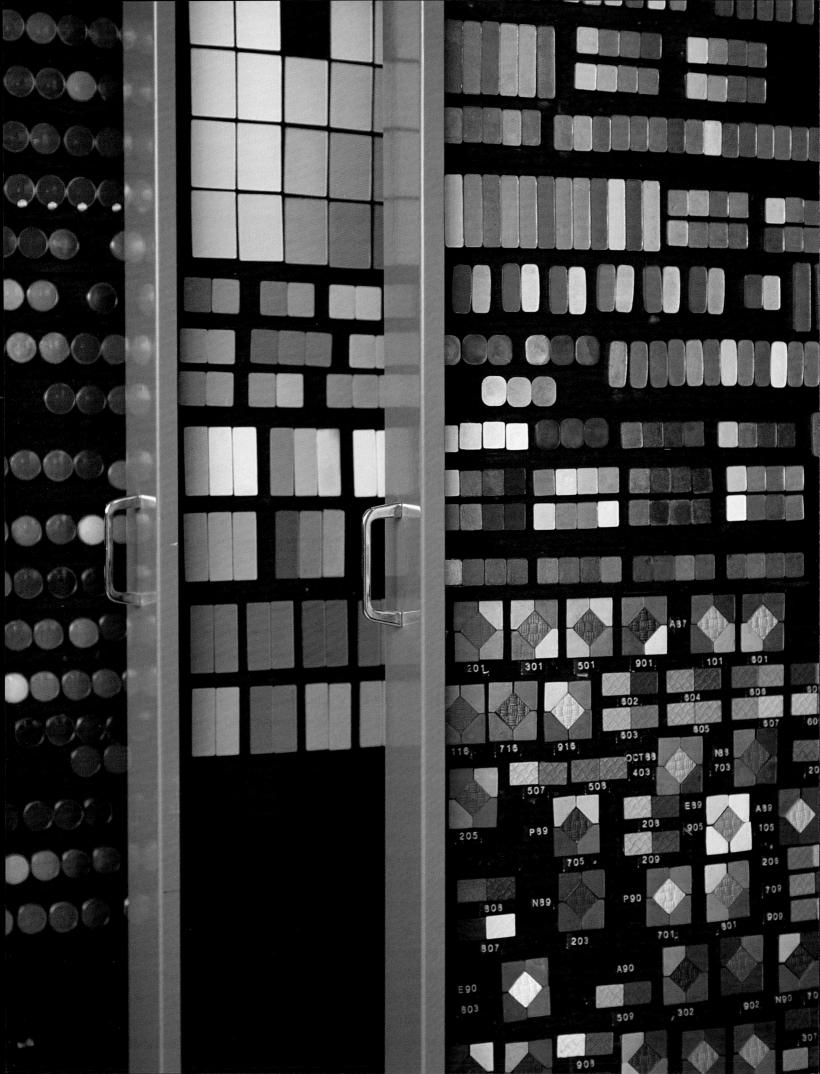

The Colors of Fashion

In the fall of 1999, Dior had 501 different shades among all its various products. And, if we are to believe Dany Sanz, quoted in *Le Monde* by Anne-Laure Quilleriet, Make Up For Ever had 1,500 products in mid-October 1998. There are far more colors than there are words to describe them. Colorists use every possible plant and flower in their descriptions, altering them with subtle nuances such as smooth, deep, saturated, unsaturated; and further modified by such qualifiers as reflections, mat, iridescent, satin, gloss, pearly. Each of these have their own shades: pinkish or more orangy. Oddly enough, nothing comes from the animal kingdom. Would this be due to the all-powerful Food and Drug Administration or the Society for the Protection of Animals? Using the name of an animal does not, however, threaten or harm it. There is "a certain green in Japan known as *yama bato iro,* the color of the mountain pigeon; in earlier times, only the mikado had the right to wear it," wrote Edmond de Goncourt in *Outamaro.* Have the feathers and plumage that surround us today become so dull that they no longer provide us with any viable examples?

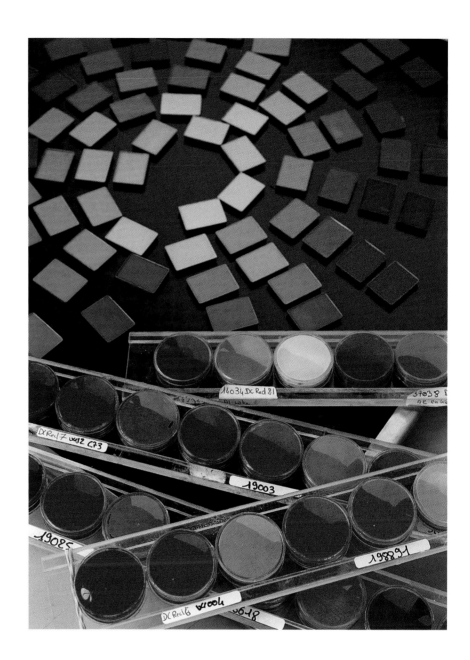

Painted from life

Dior: blocks of pigments and eyeshadow samples. Right: the Diorific Range. Left: Samples of Dior's history, with some of the 1,500 shades created by Annie Raynal for Dior: compact eyeshadow (1969–1992), and lipstick testers (1990).

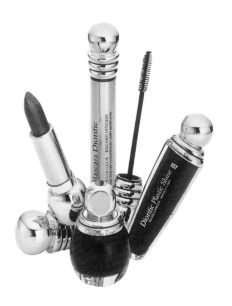

Right: The style of the moment, interpreted by a designer, from which a cosmetic "look" is created. "All the shades must be selected in harmony, therefore at the same time. A shade cannot exist alone; no more than can a single note of music. A look is like a musical score." Annie Raynal, director of Création Couleur, Parfums Christian Dior, from 1965 to 2000.

Our colors have lost some of their animal nature, as well as some of their brilliance. A product line includes colors for the face and others intended for the display case: the most audacious shades are placed prominently to attract the customer toward the trays and to inspire journalists writing in fashion magazines, yet everyone knows that these colors are rarely worn. "We are still in the middle of the 'environmental' trend," is a common complaint heard among the colorists. "Four years ago, we heard that red was on its way back in style, but we rarely see it, it doesn't sell. We have remained in the brown tones, along with the bordeaux, coppers and pinkish beiges . . ."

Is the world losing its colors? Each season, Dior takes nearly one-third of its shades off the market—this figure varies, of course, with the five or six regions of the world where the products are sold—but they are instantly replaced by others. Make-up, however, would truly have lost its color if red were to disappear.

"The charm of this paint," said Casanova, "lies in the negligence with which it is applied to the cheeks. One would not want this red to appear natural; it is daubed on to please the eye, which sees evidence of a drunkeness that holds a promise of slackened morals and enchanting passion."

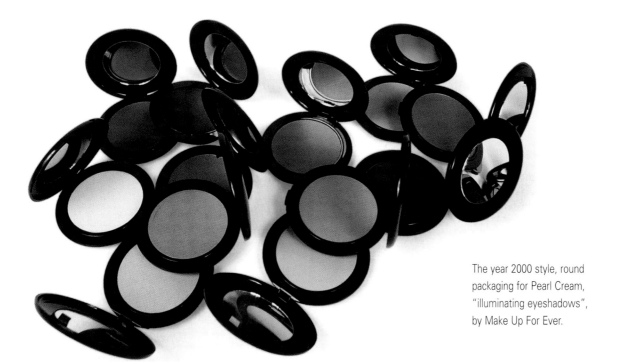

The year 2000 style, round packaging for Pearl Cream, "illuminating eyeshadows", by Make Up For Ever.

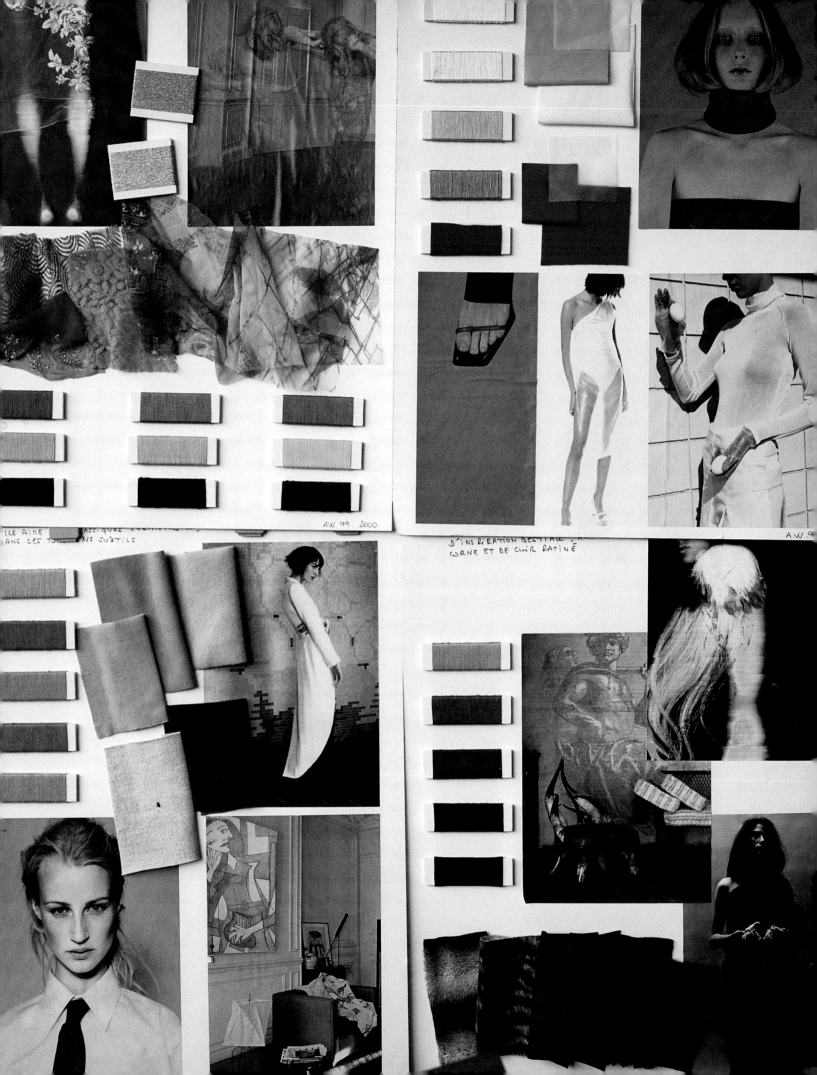

AW 99 2000

ILE AINE
ANS DES TO... RIS SUBTILS

D'INSPIRATION BESTIALE
CORNE ET DE CUIR PATINÉ

A.W.9

The complexion

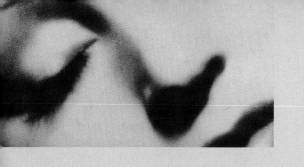

the red and
    the white

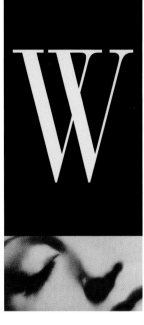

W

Women have many choices to make when it comes to their facial coloring. The extreme pallor of white skin suggests confinement, illness and death, while red symbolizes activity, youth and health. Looked at in another way, however, white skin echoes the smoothness, uniformity and perfection of a statue—art, in other words—while red can make a woman look too ruddy, raw and natural. This is the first paradox.

In the nineteenth century, this paradox was easily dealt with: since a woman's dress and the fabric it was made of were considered more important than her skin and flesh tones, the color of the skin was made to follow, if possible, that of her clothing. "With the rare feeling for harmony that characterizes them," said Théophile Gautier, "women have understood that there is a sort of dissonance between elaborate finery and a natural appearance. Just as talented painters create harmony between flesh and draperies with light-colored glazes, women lighten their skin— which would look rough next to watered silk, lace and satin—to create a unity of tone preferable to the loud white, red and pink supplied by the purest colors. Using a fine powder, they give their skin the glitter of marble by effacing its healthy ruddiness—a coarse aspect of our civilization that implies the preeminence of physical appetites over intellectual instincts. In this way, the form moves closer to statuary; women are spiritualized and purified."

The second paradox is that until the recent craze for tanning, differences in coloring served to distinguish sexes, classes and races from each other. Just because most Westerners want a good tan doesn't stop many Africans from wanting to lighten their skin.

If one of the functions of make-up is to smooth and unify the face and to create a backdrop for the designs that will be drawn on it—just as a painter prepares his canvas—then the final paradox is that only color can create the illusion of volume by

"After having described the method of cleaning and stretching the skin as well as lightening it, all that remains is to put a touch of red and vermilion in the middle of the cheeks and on the lips."
Ambroise Paré

Detail of *The Straw Hat*,
by Rubens, ca. 1622. Subtle
nuances of color beautifully
reveal the sparkle and
transparency of the complexion
and the flesh on the throat.
Preceding page:
Louise Brooks in 1928.

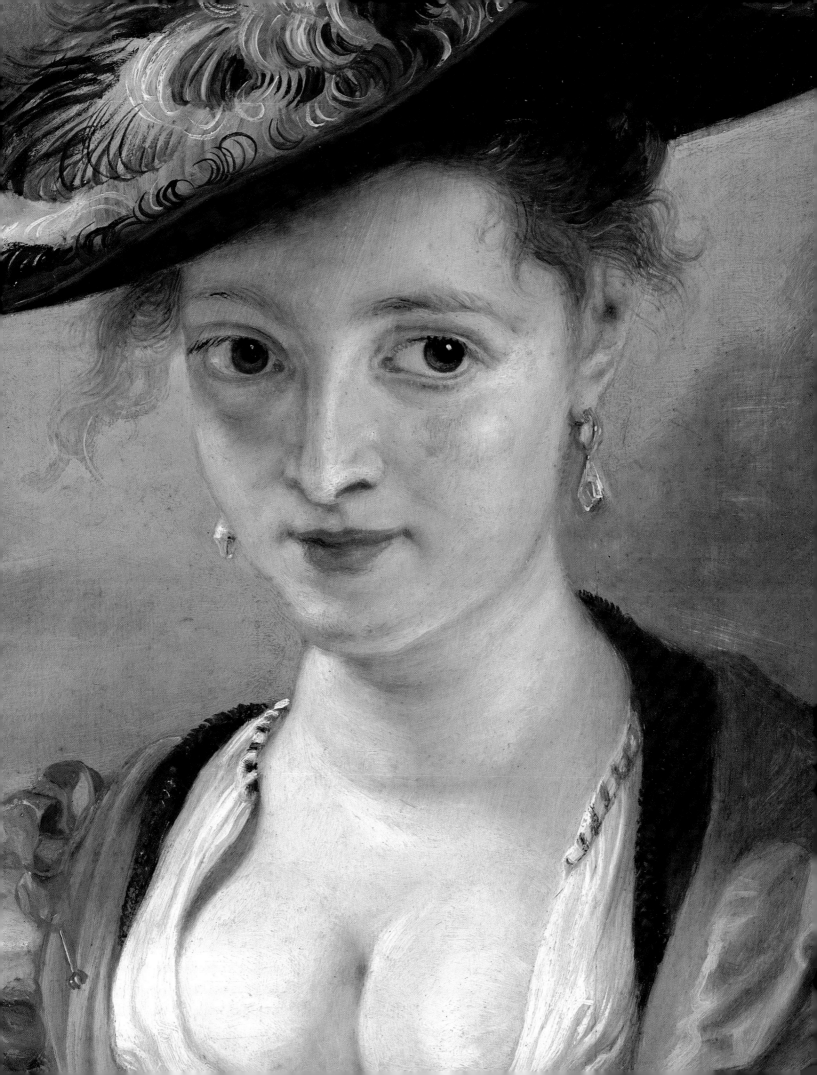

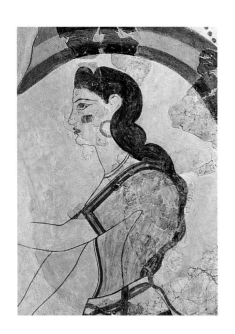

Fresco from Thera,
one of the Cyclades
islands. The fire from
the islands' crater burns
anew on the cheeks
of the women.

sculpting and modeling; not much can be done about the shape of the eye and the mouth. The face can be sculpted by playing with shadows and light, that is, with gradations of colors, which are not as uniform as they appear to be.

Finally, in terms of surface area, the face is quite different from other body parts that are made up. For a long time, make-up was used on all the revealed parts of the upper body. Gautier wrote: "Do women cover their neck, shoulders, breasts and arms with a light veil of white powder because they have been overcome by a vague shudder of modesty and want to tone down their nudity by obscuring the warm, provocative colors of life?" Wherever there is skin, make-up can be used: for Mishima's Tenkatsu, "make-up was as extreme as that of a ballad singer, with a layer of white powder extending to the very edge of the toenails." In other words, make-up practically becomes the body, making it a sort of beauty care.

White or pink, but always camellia

In Antiquity, the goal was to be as white as possible without seeming pale, not an easy accomplishment. The fathers of the Church criticized women who used white lead to look whiter than is natural, as well as those who used alkanet to pinken their complexions. Ovid, without making a judgement, spoke of those who used art "to provide the touch of vermilion that their blood sometimes refuses them," while Marbode, the bishop of Rennes, railed against women in the twelfth century who "painted their too-ruddy cheeks with white milk." Two products were available in ancient times, according to Grillet's scholarly treatise: *psimuthion,* a natural or manufactured white lead (lead carbonate), samples of which have been found in the graves of women who lived in Attica and Corinth in the third century B.C., and *paideros,* a pinkish cream made from a variety of acanthus.

Slaves who were in charge of make-up began their work by removing the creams and beauty masks that had been applied the evening before from the forehead and cheeks. They then applied white lead—according to Pliny, the most highly prized was the variety that came from Rhodes—to the whole face, beginning with the forehead. At this point, the whitened face "sometimes resembled the walls of a sepulchre," according to Jean Chrysostome. Cover-up products were then applied with chalk, although some women preferred to follow the advice of Horace and drink an infusion of cumin, which was supposed to bleach the features.

In the nineteenth century, French physician Dr. Constantin James wrote: "It would seem that, under Augustus, as in the days of our Romantic school, a slight resemblance to a tuberculosis sufferer was able to inspire sentiments warmer than simple compassion." In the Romantic era, cumin, rather than vinegar, was used to create this effect. But Montaigne had seen worse in his day: "In Paris, who has not heard talk of a woman who has her skin peeled just to acquire a complexion fresher than that of a baby? . . . I have seen some women swallow sand or ashes and go to lengths that could ruin their stomachs just to acquire a pale complexion."

At noon on Tuesday, February 23, 1847, after she had died of tuberculosis, crowds began rushing to the home of the courtesan immortalized by Dumas under the name of Marguerite Gautier. Johannès Gros wrote: "The women were not the least passionate. All the delicate and secret paraphernalia indispensable to the painting and ornamentation of beauty was spread out there and in the boudoir, including a solid silver powder box made by Marlé, a silversmith located on the Boulevard des Italiens."

The Dame aux Camélias's favorite eau de toilette was the appropriately named Eau du Harem, which she bought from the Geslin boutique on the Boulevard des Italiens. As pretty as she was, she still used the artifice of make-up to enhance her beauty, using up to ten pots of cold cream every two months. According to Eugène Rimmel, cold cream "is a type of perfected cerate that is highly useful, especially in winter, but only a small amount should be bought at a time so that it remain as fresh as possible. The addition of glycerine to cold cream increases its beneficial effects but makes it difficult to preserve."

Advertisement for Eugène Rimmel, a member of the Arts Society of London and the Horticultural Society of London and Nice. In addition to his shop at 96 the Strand in London, there were others at 128 Regent Street and 24 Cornhill in the City, and in Paris at 17, Boulevard des Italiens.

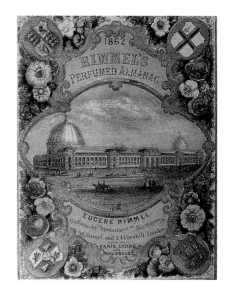

The cheeks: rouge

According to Grillet, in the fifth century B.C., there was already a Greek expression for painting the cheeks: "application of color." On a white foundation, red spots were added to the cheekbones with *phukos.* There were four or five different shades of *phukos,* depending on the variety of lichen or algae that was mixed with the fatty excipient to create a rouge of a fairly intense red, sometimes with orange highlights. *Anchousa,* a rouge made by mixing alkanet (a plant of the borage family) with a fatty excipient, was also used, as well as *miltos,* red dirt that was cheap and abundant.

A clay plate (now in the Villa Giulia Museum in Rome) found in the Etruscan city of Veii shows a frontal view of a woman's face with orange-red-colored cheekbones. A Pompeiian mosaic portrait of a woman (Museum of Naples), created by a Greek artist in the first century A.D., shows the cheekbones tinted slightly with pink. The Fayum portraits show little evidence of white lead on the cheeks, which are nearly completely colored with pink (especially *The Fayum Woman* at the Louvre).

In general, the ancient world favored pink cheeks, although the practice was neither widespread nor continuous. In Europe, Italy was the only country to retain the tradition, which was revived during the Renaissance. Finally, France, too, began to blush again (the Gauloises had been in the habit of adding red to cheeks that had been coated with chalk dissolved in vinegar), followed by all the countries subject to its influence. The rouge used was "highly colored, highly exaggerated on the day of the presentation to the court," noted Baudelaire, who mentions the portraits of Nattier as an example, "in which it blazes."

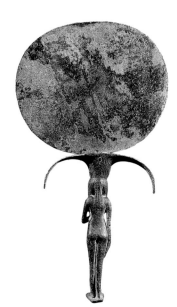

Bronze mirror with a handle in the form of a naked girl, Palestine, first or second century.
Facing page: Portrait of a woman in encaustic on wood, Fayum, Middle Egypt, second to fifth centuries. During the Roman era, these mummy portraits replaced the masks used during the Pharaonic era. Some six hundred are known and, as they are all very different, are thought to be realistic.

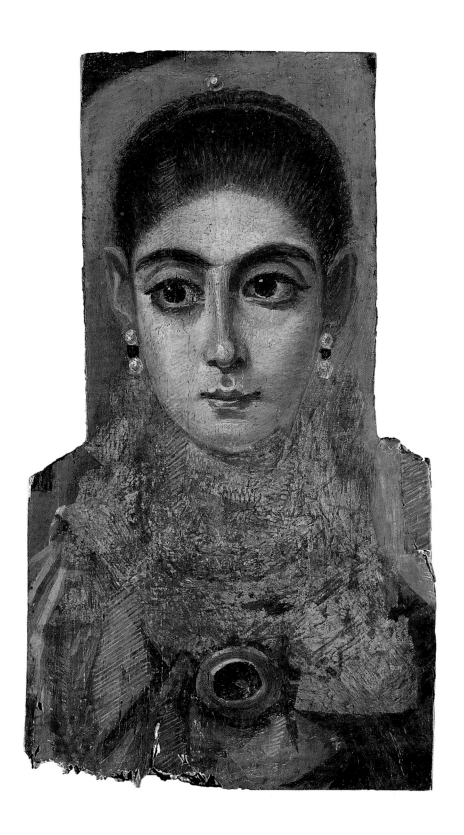

Cheeks. Those of today's women are so well disguised that they cannot even be seen properly.

Blushing. Many women blush only with the aid of a make-up brush. What is even stranger is that men also color their cheeks with rouge to make themselves look fresh and healthy. The effeminate Orore is one of them. He wouldn't think of going out without looking like one of those dolls that are the latest fashion and provide amusement to children.

Vermilion. The vermilion used by women looks more like cattle blood than anything else. That is why Blérine, who had a face like an angel before she painted her cheeks and chin scarlet, looks like a shrew.

Others imitate her, however, and already the young Clayrus paints his face and is not ashamed to borrow from the sexual organs the artifice that dishonors him and understandably makes him a laughing stock.

Caraccioli's Dictionary

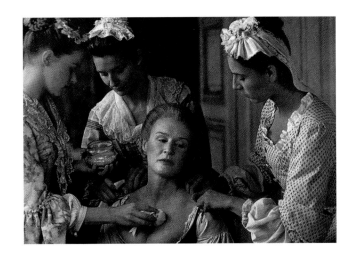
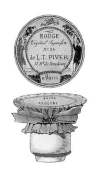
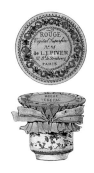

The complexion

Glenn Close in
Stephen Frears's *Dangerous
Liaisons*, with L.T. Piver's
plant-based rouge.
Facing page:
Madame Adélaïde, detail,
1756. The third daughter
of Louis XV and Marie
Leczinska, she was called
Madame Dish Rag by her
father, but you wouldn't
know it from this painting
by Nattier.

French rouge

In Stephen Frears's movie *Dangerous
Liaisons,* one of the characters
promises Valmont some rouge as a
reward for conquering Madame de
Tourvel. That might seem like a
small reward, and it is not what was
offered in the novel, in which the
Marquise de Merteuil offers herself
as the prize. But this is neither
anachronistic nor incongruous: in the
eighteenth century, people were
mad about rouge, and it was sold for
ridiculously high prices.

French rouge had a near
monopoly in Europe, and at the time
France sold two million pots of rouge
per year, according to Pinset.
Said the Baroness of Oberkirch:
"The smallest pot cost a louis,
and to obtain one that was out of
the ordinary, you had to pay
between sixty and ninety livres."
These were the prices in
Mademoiselle Martin's Temple

boutique. "Her rouge was
incontestably superior to all
the others, and one had to pay
the price."

Mademoiselle Martin was a
partner of the Martin brothers,
inventors of a varnish that carried
their name; this was an imitation of
the Japanese and Chinese lacquers
that were at the height of fashion
under the reign of Louis XV. Their
factory, a supplier to the king,
produced remarkable products for
nearly fifty years: paneling for
apartments, coaches, furniture and
jewelry of all sorts. The connection
with rouge helps to explain
Caraccioli's expression, "to blush like
the wheel of a coach": "At the
beginning of the century, a timid
brush trembled when applied to the
face and seemed to regret adding a
trace of red to it, but since the
Duchess of . . . became the first to
dare to blush like the wheel of a

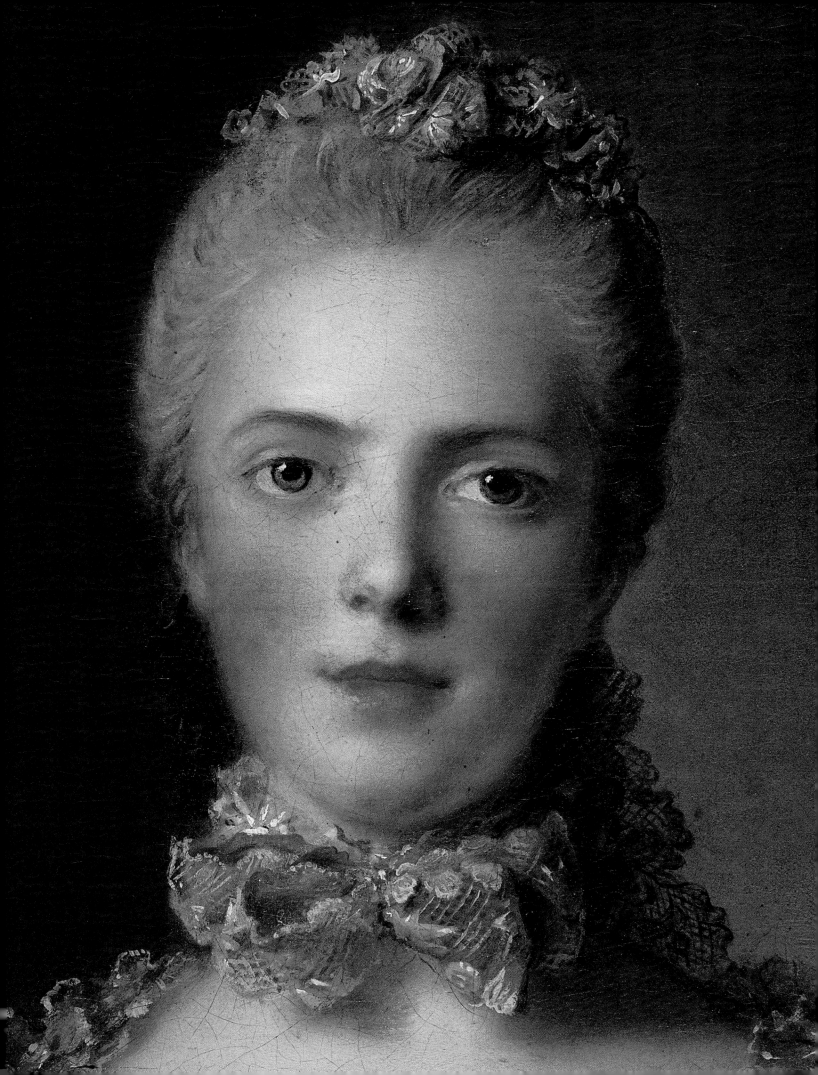

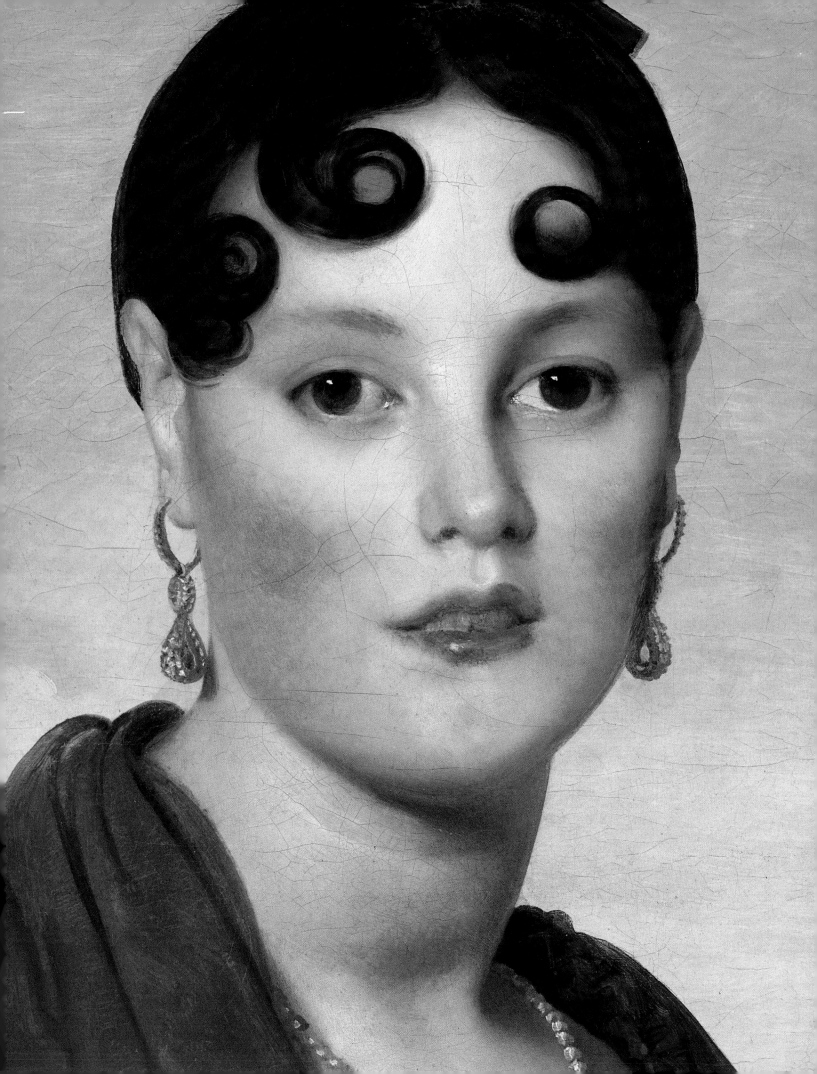

coach, ladies' bedrooms resemble painters' studios. Women are not content to appear bright red; they want to be crimson. . . . Mademoiselle Martin had cornered the high end of the market: she had the queen's patent as well as those of all the female royals of Europe. . . . She had permission to have pots made in Sèvres just for her, and she sent them to the queens; hardly any duchesses were able to obtain them. We were highly amused by her importance." These pots are among the finest and best decorated porcelains from Vincennes and Sèvres.

Fréderik, a women's hairdresser located on the Rue Thibautodé (off the Quai de la Mégisserie) in Paris, "supplied a Portuguese rouge known for the finesse and softness of its nuance." Houbigant, located on Paris's Faubourg Saint-Honoré in 1775 in a boutique called La Corbeille de Fleurs, "makes and sells perfumes, plant-based rouge, gloves

and fans," according to his brochure. Balzac, like the characters in his *Human Comedy,* would be one of the shop's customers in the following century.

In London and Venice, and at the small courts of Germany, Constantinople and Saint Petersburg, the arrival of the "Poupée de France" and French rouge was eagerly awaited. Occasionally, someone couldn't bear to wait; the Duke de Gotha paid a secretary whose only job was to keep him informed, month by month, of developments in Parisian elegance, one of which was the latest method of applying rouge and beauty spots. In Weimar, Goethe wrote plays for princes' huge birthday parties, to which all who had the same first name as the sovereign were invited. A military parade, theater gala and banquet were held at each party, and the women wore a spot of rouge on their faces.

Rouge by Bourjois: the first dry rouge for the theater (top), 1863, and one of the first rouges for everyday wear, Rosette Brune, 1879. Facing page: *La Belle Zélie,* a portrait of Madame Aymon by Ingres, detail, 1806. "Mr. Ingres loves color like a shopkeeper loves fashion," wrote Baudelaire.

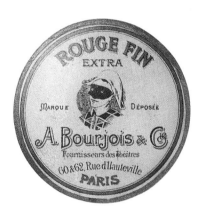

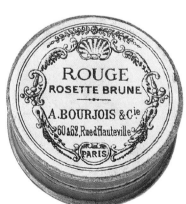

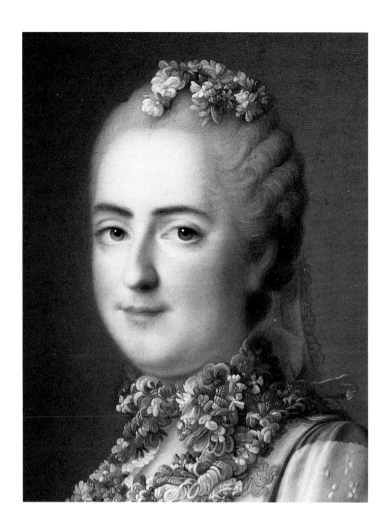

Portrait of Madame Louise
(detail), sister of Adélaïde
and a future Carmelite
nun at Saint-Denis. Studio
of F.-H. Drouais.

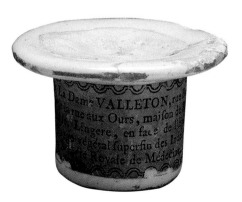

Pot of rouge from the
Fragonard perfumery,
eighteenth century.
Facing page: Can you spot
Mozart in *The Wedding of
Joseph II and Isabella of Parma*
(detail), by Martin Meytens,
now in Vienna's Schönbrunn
Palace? Hint: the marriage took
place on October 16, 1760,
when the composer was four
years old.

Red as a poppy

There was no sense in applying
rouge in private, since it was
obviously an artifice. The fact that a
woman used make-up was no longer
a secret. Count de Vaublanc
reported: "No matter where they
were, many women openly touched
up their pretty red cheeks in public."
No attempt made to be discreet: "At
Versailles, the court princesses wear
it bright and demand the same of
the others present," wrote the
Goncourt brothers. Rouge was a
matter of etiquette and official
protocol. The pious Marie Leczinska,
wife of Louis XV, always had
difficulty with it, yet when it turned
out that Maria Teresa of Spain, who
in 1745 married her oldest son, the
dauphin Louis, didn't use make-up, it
created a diplomatic scandal that had
to be defused by the Duke of
Richelieu. Seven years later, their
daughter Henriette, the king's
favorite, was made up on her death
bed. "She was," said Barbier in his
diary, "laid out on a mattress,
wearing a bed jacket and rouge."

When Marilyn Monroe died, her
lawyers, to whom she had given
specific orders, called her personal
make-up artist, Whity, in New York.
True to his promise, he jumped on a
plane, taking his fiancée, a
hairdresser, with him. During the trip
and until they arrived at the hospital,
they drank to give themselves

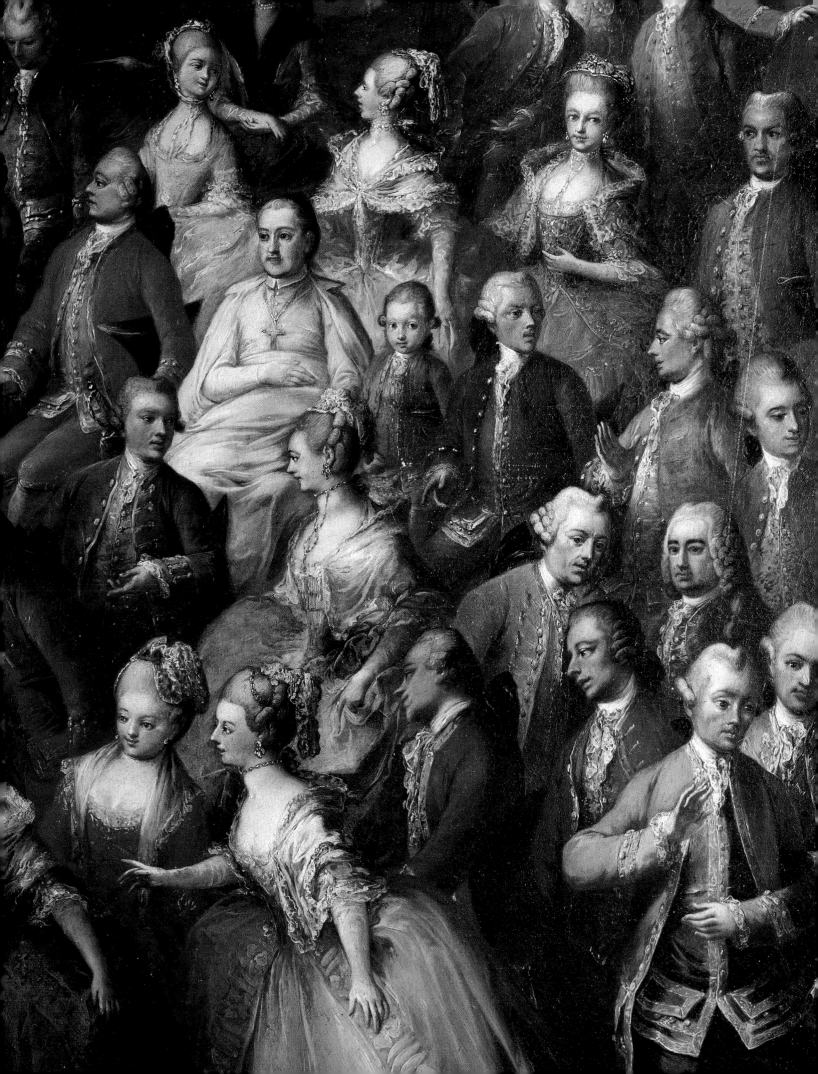

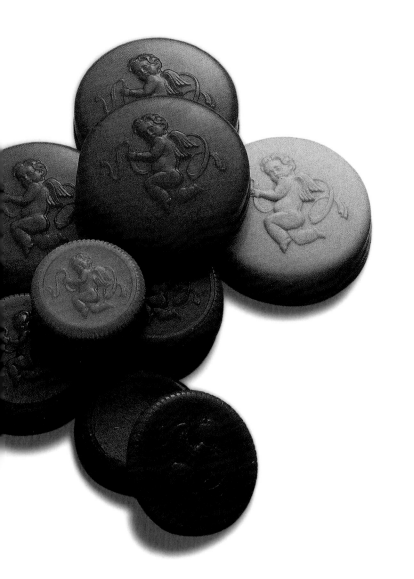

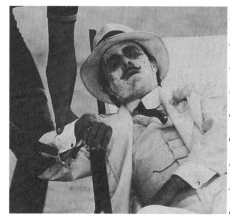

Dirk Bogarde plays
Aschenbach in
Luchino Visconti's film of
Death in Venice, 1970.
Above: An angel watches
over rouge by Lancôme.

A fight to the death

In 1883, Pierre Loti was an officer aboard the cruiser Atalante, *which was on its way to Tonkin. One of his comrades, Jean Desrieux, described him as having "a hard face, like a knife blade, brush-cut hair and a stiff mustache cut even with the lips. He did not wear rice powder, in spite of what has been said, but a few touches of carmine on the lips and a glaze of pink on the cheekbones, which brought out the tanned patina of his coloring."*

At the end of 1896, he was the commander of the Javelot. *Francis Jammes described him during a gala held in the Basque country: "His long nose stuck out between his painted cheekbones and in his round, wide eyes an abyss opened onto who knows what dark night. They showed compassion and fear and made you forget the cloud of make-up."*

Loti himself said: "We must protect ourselves against old age. We have no right to become an object of disgust."

In Death in Venice, *Thomas Mann says of his character Aschenbach: "In comparison with the delicious adolescent he was smitten with, his aging body disgusted him. Seeing his gray hair and the deep lines on his face, he was overcome with shame and despair. Something pushed him to make his body fresh again, to redo it."*

Later, he adds, "Lower, where once the skin was flabby, yellowish and wrinkled, Aschenbach saw a slight blush appear: his lips, bloodless minutes ago, took on a raspberry tone; the wrinkles on his cheeks and lips, and the crow's feet around his eyes disappeared under the cream and the rejuvenating lotion . . . With a pounding heart, Aschenbach discovered a blooming adolescent in the mirror."

courage. Then he made Marilyn up and she did her hair to make her beautiful one last time.

Rouge on the cheeks is a sign of life. Lola Montès had an expression to describe people ill with what today we would call stress or simply old age, "Losing one's roses": "A little plant-based rouge on the cheeks of a beautiful woman, who, because of bad health or a troubled spirit, is losing her roses, is excusable, and the texture of this rouge is so transparent (if it is not adulterated with lead) that, when the blood rises to the face, it speaks, even if it is a thin layer, and brings out the bloom on a fading cheek."

To carry signs of life until death is to continue to live. It was the blush on her cheeks that saved Snow White: because her beautiful cheeks were still red, the dwarves didn't bury her and simply laid her out in what was more a box than a casket, from which she would be awakened, according to differing versions of the story, by a jolt or a kiss. With her red cheeks, complexion as white as snow and hair black as ebony, Snow White is the incarnation of make-up and the personification of three colors. The way she is depicted in different eras marks a historic shift

in the use of make-up: In the 1812 Grimm Brothers' version, her cheeks were as red as blood; in the 1937 Walt Disney version, her lips were as red as roses.

At that time, Elizabeth Arden wrote: "Apply your rouge when your face is still slightly damp by tapping lightly with the tips of the fingers. Liquid rouge should be applied with the help of a small cotton wad soaked in Tonique (at first, apply only small quantities at a time and continue in this way until you have acquired experience). Spread the rouge gently, shading the contours. Don't put it too close to the eyes or the nose, otherwise you will have a too bright, unnatural look. It is better to put on too little than too much. Now, put on powder."

In Europe, the process was exactly the opposite in the eighteenth century: "Good taste requires that rouge be very heavy, that it touch the lower eyelids. They say that this gives fire to the eyes," said Count de Vaublanc. We have seen that Laclos agreed, as did Baudelaire: "Rouge, which inflames the cheekbone, increases the clarity of the pupil and adds the mysterious passion of a priestess to a beautiful female face."

A 1927 advertisement for Bourjois. It appeared in the *Annuaire du Couturier Paul Poiret,* among others.

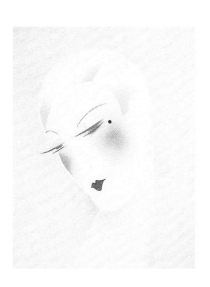

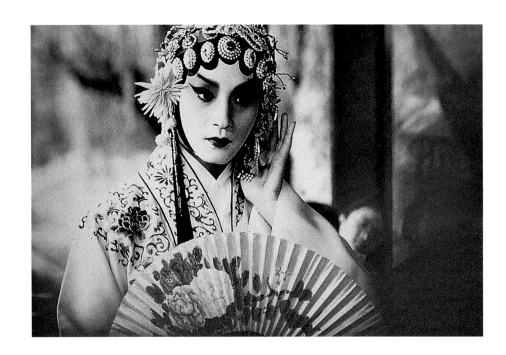

The actor Leslie Cheung,
trained to play women's roles
in the Peking Opera,
in Chen Kaige's film
Farewell My Concubine, 1993.

Creating a
healthy look

These differing approaches require
us to choose between the eyes and
the complexion. Rouge may make
the eyes smolder, but the rest of the
face seems yellowish in comparison.
"The presence of heavy rouge
yellows all that is around it," says
Diderot's *Encyclopédie*. "One
resigns oneself to being yellow, and
that is surely not the color of
beautiful skin."

Helena Rubinstein's response:
"We do not resign ourselves to
being yellow, and to avoid this, it is
enough to not limit rouge to the
cheeks. Make-up on the cheeks
makes you look younger and
healthier. If you look tired, drawn,
slightly sunken, put a very light
touch of rouge on the middle and
sides of the forehead and on the
temples. Spread the color by shading
it toward the corner of the eyes to
join the brighter spot that you have
put on your cheeks, then spread it up
to the hairline. You will have a superb
look even if you feel exhausted."

Make-up has been "natural" for a
long time. It is used to restore natural
colors when they have been
accidentally altered; this could be
called maintenance and restoration
make-up. Gone are the days when no
attempt was made to hide the fact that
one was wearing rouge, when a
woman chose her coloring as she
would choose her outfit, according to
the circumstances, place, season, and
her status and rank. "The appalling
mistresses of butcher's boys wear
rouge . . . the color of blood; the trashy
courtesans of the Palais-Royal wear
rouge the color of roses. . . . Women
at court, who play for high stakes, pay

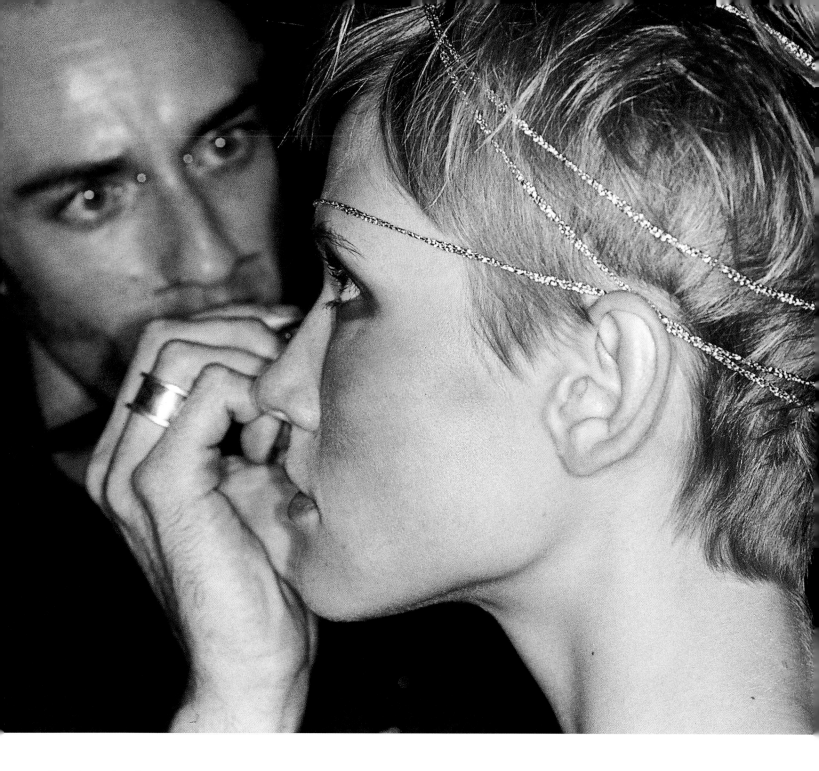

The make-up artist and
his model in Julien
McDonald's salon during
London Fashion Week, 1998.

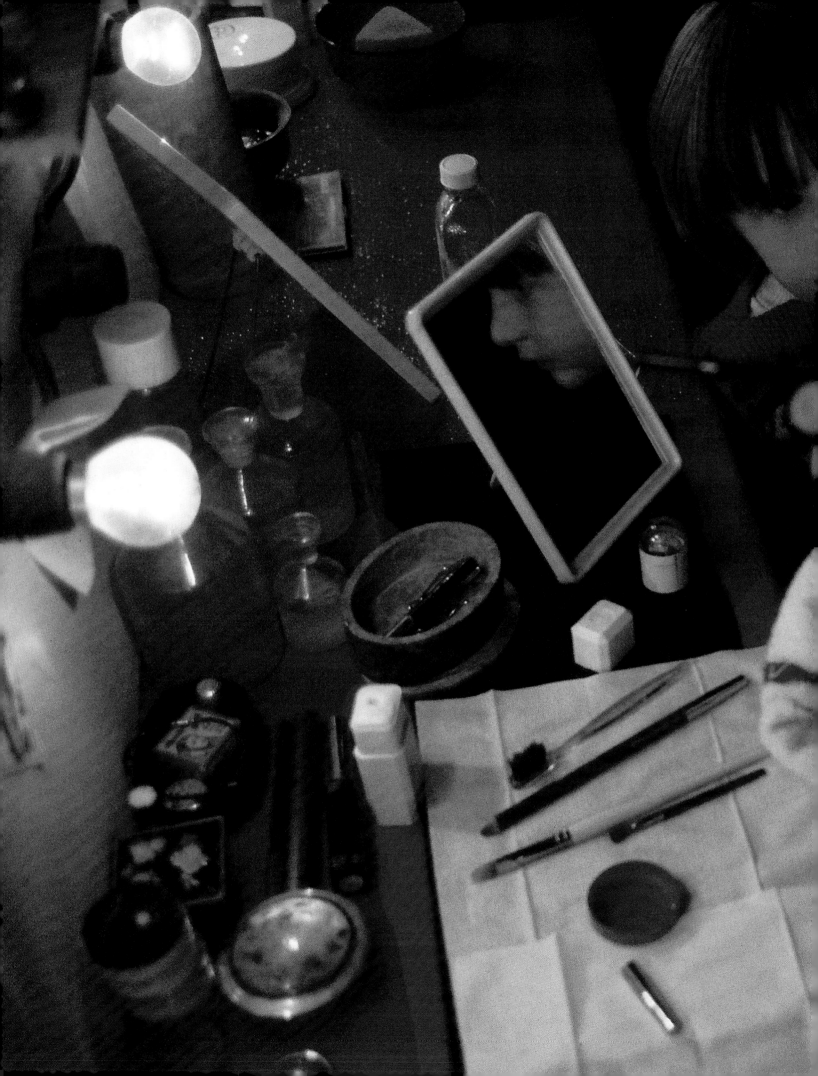

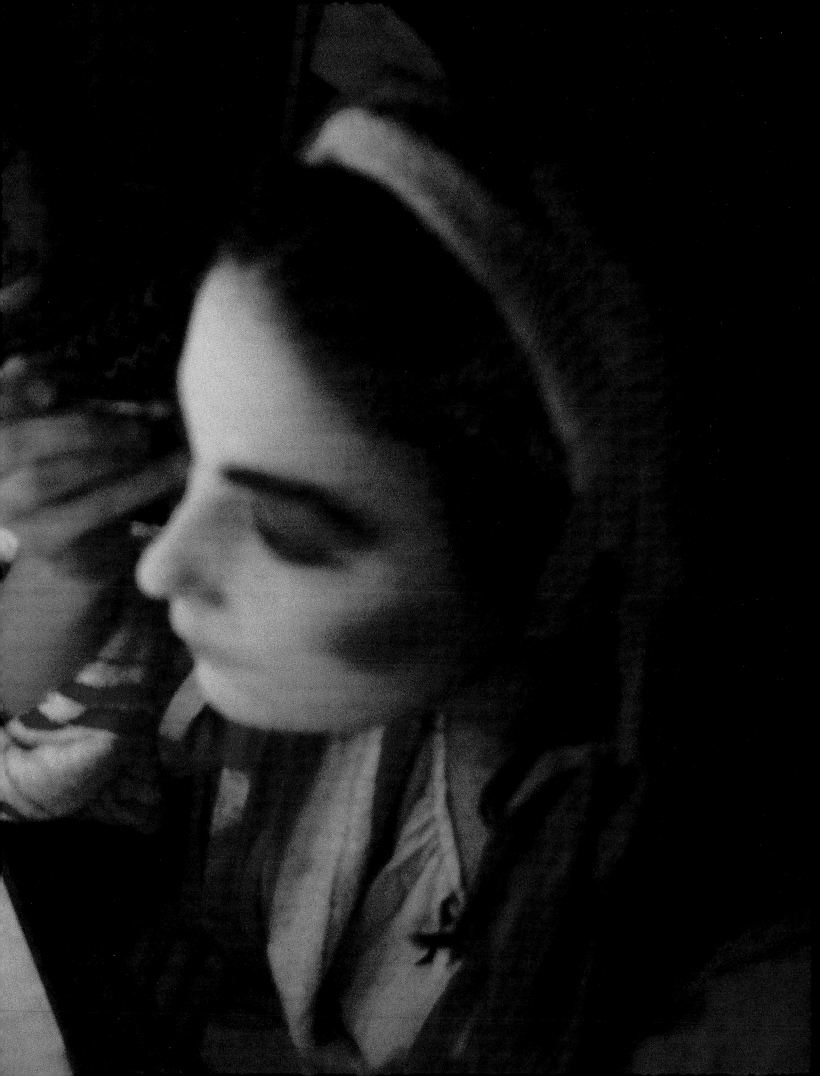

The complexion

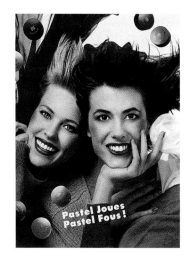

Pastel Joues
Pastel Fous!

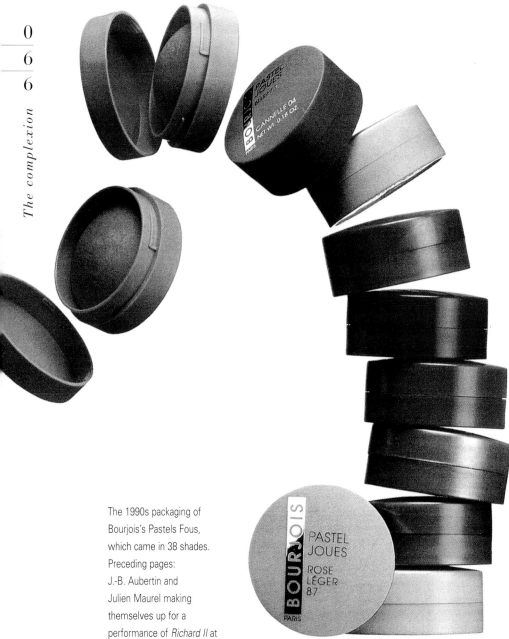

BOURJOIS
PARIS
PASTEL
JOUES
ROSE
LÉGER
87

The 1990s packaging of
Bourjois's Pastels Fous,
which came in 38 shades.
Preceding pages:
J.-B. Aubertin and
Julien Maurel making
themselves up for a
performance of *Richard II* at
the Théâtre du Soleil, 1982.

a louis for a small pot; women of quality pay twelve francs; and middle-class women, who put on imperceptible amounts, don't bargain for it."

Conspicuous rouge was worn all over the world. In China, heavy rouge was applied in two carefully marked circles just under the eyes for five centuries, from the seventh to eleventh centuries, under the Tang and Northern Song dynasties. And, more recently, according to Rimmel, Chinese women "colored their cheeks, lips, nostrils and the tip of the tongue with cochineal spread on little cards whose green metallic surface turned bright red when the finger was wet." Japanese women "coated their faces with white lead and colored the cheeks and lips with safflower. They sometimes exaggerated the dose so much that their coloring was purple."

The bayaderes (professional dancers) of India "covered their cheeks with rouge when they were very pale. To obtain rouge of this color, they had only to mix a little quicklime and grated yellow nut sedge in water; the yellow plant soon turned dark red." In Tahiti, Queen Pomaré wore rouge on her cheeks, according to Admiral Dupetit-Thouars.

The decline of rouge

Eventually, wearing conspicuous rouge became an embarrassment. It was also toxic (though less so than white lead), and even when it was made of sandalwood or brazilwood, it still contained sulfur or mercury. The hygienic nineteenth century leaned toward healthier Oriental products: "As little inclined as we are to admit the superiority of these cosmetics (kohl as a remedy for ophthalmia and henna, which is supposed to cure cracked skin), we must nevertheless make an exception for *schnouda,* which women use to brighten the colors of their complexion. This cream, which is composed of sublimated benzoin, acts as a mild stimulant on the skin, lending it perfectly natural colors for a few hours without the drawbacks that are rightly attributed to European rouge."

Beginning with the Second Empire, the evolution of rouge can be traced on Bourjois's round rouge containers: first, the product was called just "Theatrical Rouge," but later the qualification "approved by the medical schools of Paris," was added to the packaging. Then it was referred to as being for everyday rather than theatrical use, and the company A. Bourjois & Cie, "theatrical supplier," became a "special maker of products for the beauty of ladies." After World War I, the masked harlequin of its beginnings was replaced by garlands of flowers, then by Venus looking into a mirror on a vase inspired by Antiquity, then by an imitation shagreen box in the same color as its contents and engraved with its name: Mandarin Red, Apricot Red, Dusty Pink, Dusty Purple, etc. By this time, the company had an entire range of products, which took on a touch of exoticism at the end of the 1920s with names like Rajah Ocher, Yeddah Ocher, etc.

In the mid-1930s, Elizabeth Arden's rouge was available in eleven shades. "When it is applied with skill, it has a very natural look and stays on all day. Red Head is perfect for those with light skin, who often have Venetian blond hair. The Chariot, Victoire and Coquette rouges harmonize with the lipsticks of the same tones. Geranium G. is for blonds, and Sunburn rouge is for suntanned complexions. Rose Color Venetian, a clear liquid rouge, should be used on fine, 'transparent' skin." But why even use rouge if the goal is that it should not be seen?

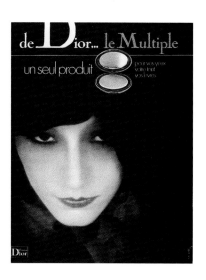

Serge Lutens created the Multiple line of make-up for Dior in the spring-summer season of 1974.

The skin: white

In 1798, François Gérard's painting *Cupid and Psyche* put an end to the use of rouge and brought back into fashion the pallor that was thought to be typical of Antiquity. Women began to make themselves up to look like Psyche. It would still be some time before suntanned skin became fashionable; this didn't happen until sun creams and bathing suits with removable straps came along around 1930 to enable "a uniform tan." At that time, Elizabeth Arden offered Velva Beauty Film, a matte make-up for the shoulders, arms and legs that did not stain clothing; it came in eggshell, dark, evening and suntan shades. A suntan oil facilitated a two-tone tan—coffee- and honey-colored—to create a "very pretty sports make-up."

Twenty years earlier, one of Helena Rubinstein's first New York advertisements was still saying, "You can avoid a tanned look and freckles. If your delicate skin suffers from being exposed to the sun, H.R. will provide you with an effective way of avoiding this annoyance." In the United States, even in the northeast, the absolute ideal was still that of *Gone with the Wind:* ". . . Her magnolia-white skin so prized by Southern women and so carefully guarded by bonnets, veils and mittens against hot Georgia suns."

We have just looked at a few protective methods, but human beings had been using others for some time. The first was shelter: "A great lady took care to preserve the freshness of her complexion, not with a veil but by staying in the shade during the hottest hours," said French Egyptologist Christiane Desroches-Noblecourt of Egyptian women.

In the Arab world, elegant wealthy women always took care to cover their head and face to

This is not a case of art imitating life but of life imitating art: every woman wanted a face like Psyche's. Facing page: *Cupid and Psyche,* by François Gérard, detail, 1798.

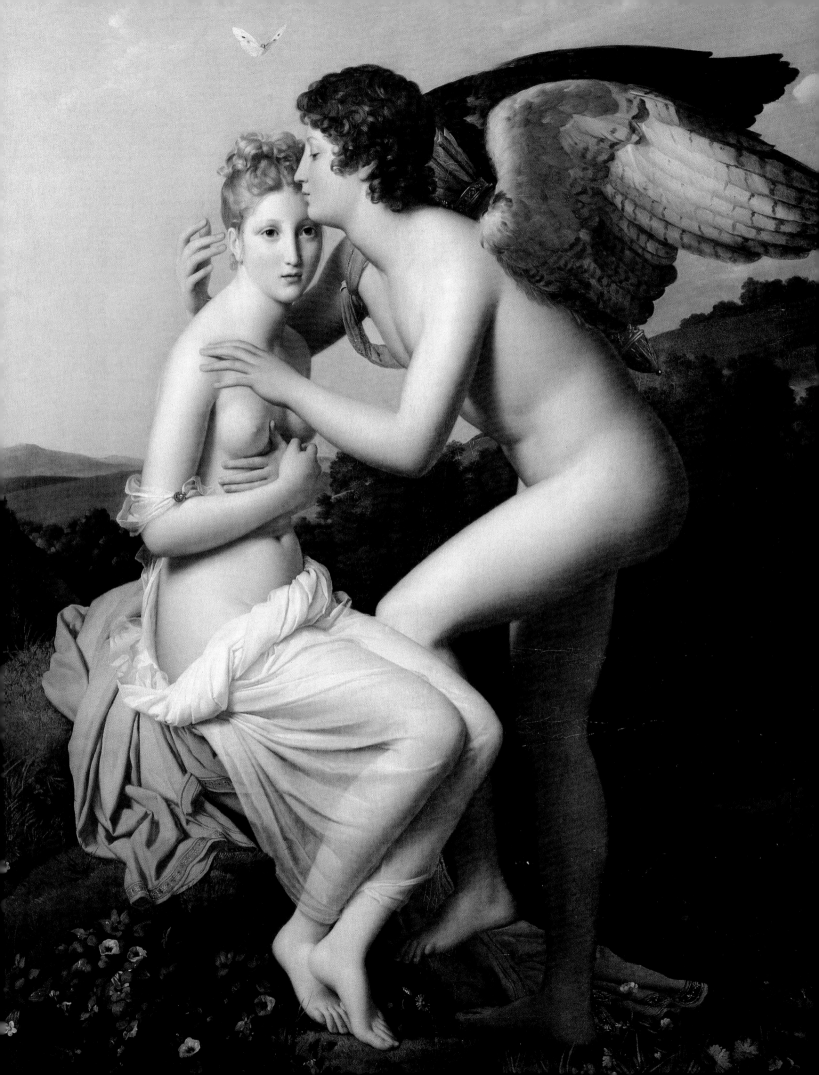

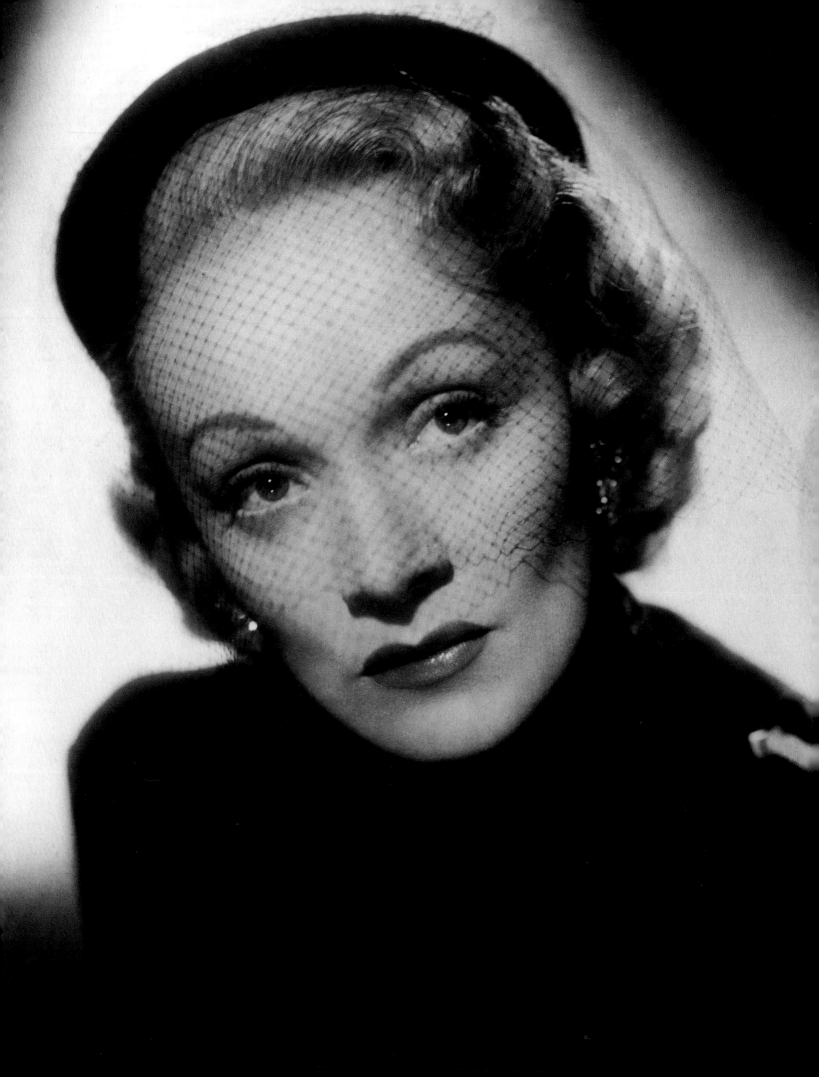

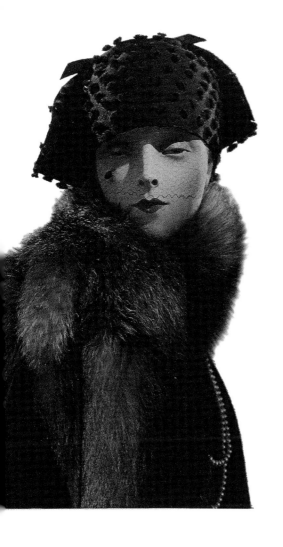

A silver fox hat by Reboux and a dress by Worth on a Siegel model, 1927. Facing page: Marlene Dietrich did her own make-up (photo: Studio Harcourt, 1939). She drew a white line along the bridge of the nose to lengthen the snub nose that displeased her. She also put white on the inside of her eyelids.

protect the freshness, smoothness and radiance of their complexions, but lower-class women were never veiled. Mohammed wanted all women to wear the veil since they were all equally noble in their faith in Allah.

In France, since the time of Charles IX, ladies of quality had been protecting their complexion from the sun by wearing a mask. Queen Elizabeth of England owned eighty wigs and almost as many masks. Under Louis XIII, the mask was the most common means of fighting the harmful effects of bad weather. The mask folded in two and was sometimes decorated with frills and flounces. Paul Scarron wrote: "Shall I speak of those capricious persons/ Who wear lace on their masks/ To bedeck the eyeholes/ Thinking that the mask is at its best."

Madame de Sévigné wrote to her daughter on June 26, 1675: "On the contrary, you must moisten the skin to freshen the complexion, and wear a mask when you go outside." Under the First Empire, women wore a veil of gauze or another light fabric when they went out. In 1900, the revue *Lectures pour tous* explained that "the effect of brisk air on the skin causes it to lose its finesse. Our readers have a simple way of remedying this inconvenience: They wear a hat veil. It is known today that this lightweight net that goes so well with the feminine face plays an important role in the protection of the complexion. M. Merlier offers two 'Coquet Minois' boxes. One contains twelve hat veils or six veils and a Chantilly scarf; the other, six veils of the latest style."

The complexion

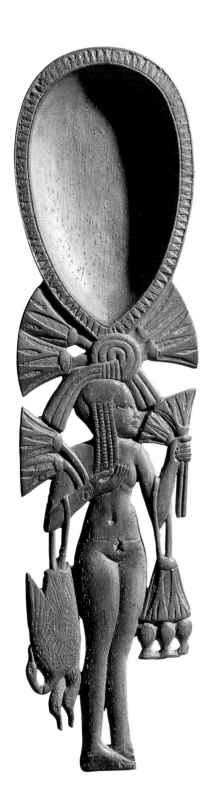

Make-up spoon dating from
the Eighteenth Dynasty,
1580–1320 B.C.
Facing page: During the
same period, King Horemheb
is depicted presenting
an offering to the goddess
Isis. The difference in
complexions, which is quite
clear here, did not distinguish
the earthly from the divine
but male from female.

A world of
pale women

For a while, it seemed as if Woman, eternally and everywhere, had a natural taste for white. The description "snow-white skin" is used in everything from texts accompanying Japanese prints to Ovid's Latin writings. For American southerners from Georgia, one might be tempted to think, however, that the most important thing was to create the strongest contrasts possible to prove without a doubt that they were radically different from the slaves on their plantations, just as aristocrats of the Classical era sought to distinguish themselves from peasants working in the fields. Islam, which expanded rapidly in the ninth century, decreed that all women should be veiled, but tens of millions of them did not wear the veil because it would have hampered them in their work. The result was that the veil became a sort of beauty accessory that distinguished a social class.

In most cases, women did not necessarily have to be white but simply have a lighter skin color than men. In Egyptian paintings, women have an ocher-yellow tint, while men are ocher-red. This applied to depictions of both humans and gods, although one would imagine that the

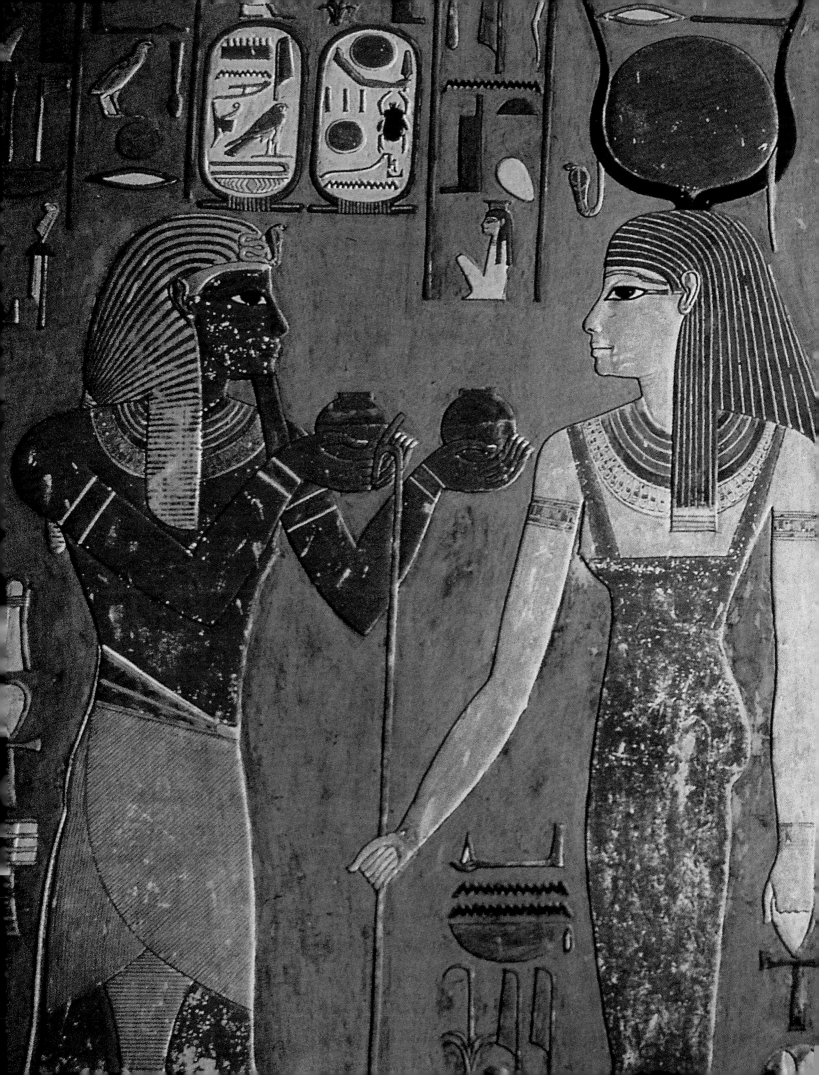

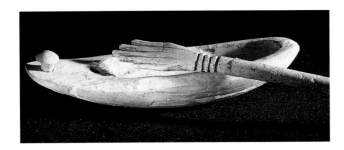

Above: Make-up container from the Hyksos period, 1730–1580 B.C. Below: An Attic vase from Epilykos, sixth century B.C. Two-and-a-half millennia later, the world moved toward one color, with some darkening their skin and others lightening it.

The complexion

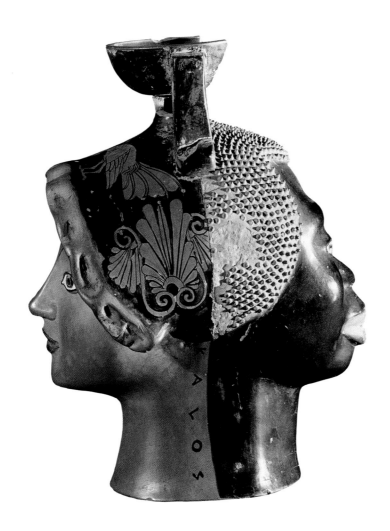

gods were less concerned with getting a suntan. The goal was to distinguish the sexes and the roles assigned to them. This is confirmed by the fact that only the goddess Hathor, who had a double nature, was depicted with dark coloring identical to that of male figures.

Among the Aztecs, according to Jacques Soustelle, "women, who naturally had dark, bronzed skin, sought a light yellow coloring, with which they are often represented in figurative manuscripts, in contrast to men. They obtained this coloring by using an ointment called *axin* or with *tecozauitl*, yellowish earth so highly prized that some provinces supplied it as tribute."

According to Haafner, who was in charge of the books of all the Dutch East Indies Company offices, in 1779, the bayaderes of India had "the custom of making themselves up, not with red or white, but with the color yellow, for which they used a particular type of yellow nut sedge, or Indian saffron, which is called *gondha-horiedra* in Sanskrit. It has a lovely golden-yellow color and a very pleasant aroma."

This type of make-up was also used by Javanese women to enhance their natural golden tint, according to Rimmel, the perfume supplier to the French emperor, the Spanish queen, the king of Portugal, the queen of Holland and the Princess of Wales. "This orangish tint is celebrated in their poetry, just as that of our ladies is compared to lilies and roses in our madrigals, and cosmetics made with saffron are very popular in this country."

The replacement of lily-white and pink complexions with suntans was the result of more than just a change in taste. It marked the beginning of an era of lack of differentiation and did, among other things, prefigure the unisex trend. But while the Western woman abandoned along with white skin all signs of distinction, some African women went in for skin lightening. Called *xessal* in Senegal and *maquillage* in Zaire and Congo, the process was effected by the same awful methods described by Jean-Luc Bonniol: "The 'burning' is done with industrial detergents, and the skin takes on a crusty appearance that is reminiscent of that of a leper or someone with a skin disease. This is followed by the second phase, 'planing,' designed to remove dead skin and smooth the epidermis. The whitening can then begin, based on the action of cortisone-based products (dermatological creams) or hydroquinone (cosmetic). On her wedding day, the young woman comes out of seclusion, lightened and 'beautified'."

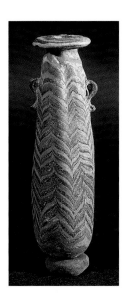

An alabaster (because they were at first made of alabaster) from Morocco, sixth century B.C. The neck was narrow and the rim flat so that the perfume would spread.

One of Ovid's recipes: "Even though incense is pleasing to the gods and calms their wrath, we must not burn it all on the braziers of their temples. Mix incense with niter to cover pimples on the skin, using four ounces of each. Add one-quarter less of gum from tree bark and a piece of myrrh the size of a die. After the mixture has been ground, put it through a sieve and thin the resulting powder with honey. Some women like to add fennel to the odorous myrrh; nine measures of myrrh require five of fennel. Add a handful of dried roses, sal ammoniac and strong incense. The weight of the sal ammoniac and the incense should equal that of the roses. Pour in an infusion of barley. When your skin is rubbed with this cosmetic, it will immediately shine with the most pleasant colors."

Another of his recipes reads: "Remove the straw and the husk from the barley that your vessels have carried from the fields of Libya. Take two pounds of this hulled barley; add an equal amount of ers (hybrid lentils) and soak it in ten eggs. When the ingredients have dried in the air, have them ground by a she-ass on a millstone." Today, the milling can be accomplished by more rapid electric means. For the ingredients, we also need two ounces of grated buck's antler, twelve crushed narcissus bulbs, two ounces of gum and of Tuscan spelt, and nine times as much honey.

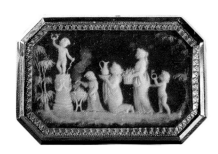

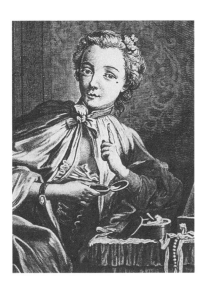

In the eighteenth century, applying a beauty spot was part of the ritual of an elegant person's toilette.
Above: *Woman Applying Beauty Spots,* after François Boucher.
Top: Gold beauty spot box, ca. 1779, Musée des Arts Décoratifs. On the cover is a bas-relief in the style of a cameo.

Beauty spots and blue blood

White is white only in contrast to another color. Scarlett O'Hara was accompanied by her mammy, and, in the world of painting, Rubens' Venus had the slave who tends her hair and Nicolas Regnier's courtesan had the "Diseuse de Bonne Aventure," just two of innumerable examples in painting. For ordinary mortals who must go it on their own, the contrasting role is played by the beauty spot. The Duchess of Mazarin continued to wear one even when she went to live in retirement with the nuns of Sainte-Marie. An effort has always been made to erase any irregularities, the slightest accident, the smallest imperfection on our skin, which is meant to be as smooth and even as possible. Many battles have been fought against redness and, worse, birthmarks. And just when uniformity was achieved, black beauty marks or blue veins were added.

In Pharaonic Egypt, "texts tell us (there are no examples in artworks) that the veins of the face were traced in blue," wrote Pinset. From Propertius's ninth *Elegy,* in which it is asked whether a woman improves her coloring by rubbing the temples with indigo, Rimmel deduces that the blue served simply to define the veins on the forehead and temples. In France, the color blue helped the aristocracy conspicuously show off its blue blood. Mercier describes the phenomenon in his *Tableau de Paris,* and, at the end of the nineteenth century, Doctor James wrote that "some women use it as an obligatory complement to the decoration of their person. Blue make-up is made with talcum reduced to an extremely fine powder, tinted in the desired proportion with Prussian blue, then transformed into a paste by the addition of slightly gummy water. Once the paste is dry, it is made into sticks or put into historiated pots like other make-up. Applicators made of goatskin are sold expressly for this purpose. You dip this point in your blue and delicately trace the veins as if you were tracing a drawing." The veins also had to remain visible through white make-up.

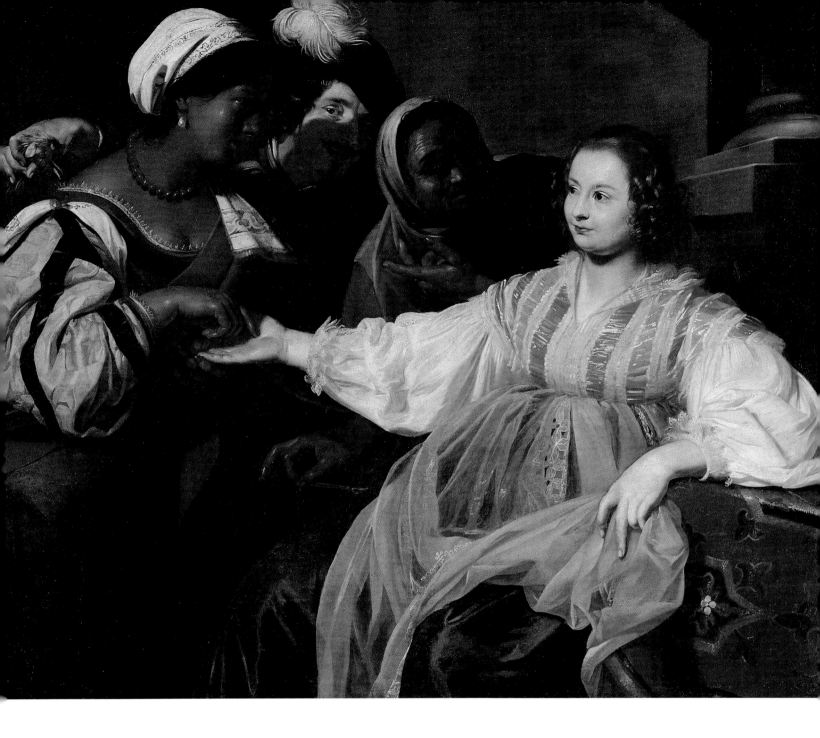

This courtesan is white, glowing,
phosphorescent. Make-up
has turned her into a beacon.
Above: *The Fortune-Teller,* by
Nicolas Régnier, 1624–1625.
Right: An exceptional piece belonging
to the collection of the Musée des
Arts Décoratifs, this beauty spot box
(ca. 1789) has three compartments.
It is made of gold with enamel
decoration and is inset with diamonds;
the brush has a gold handle.

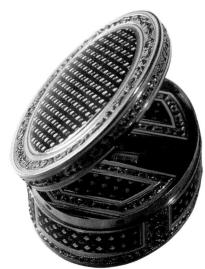

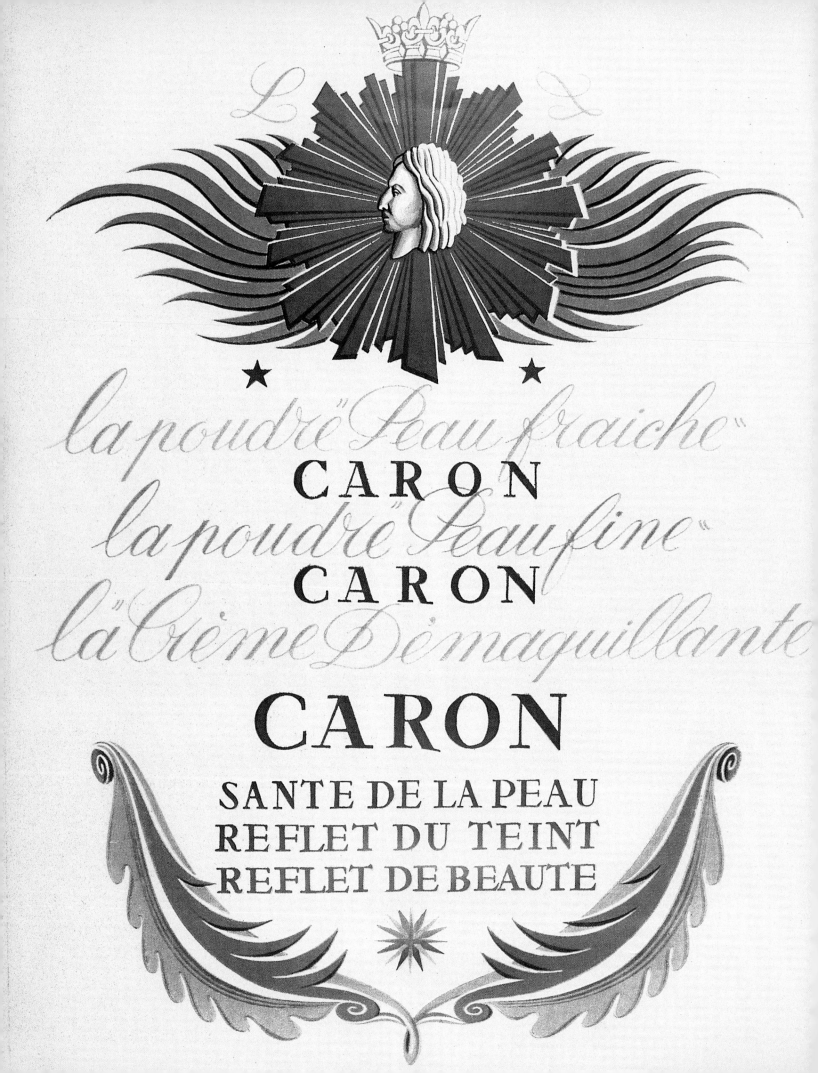

The complexion and health care

A person's facial coloring is the same as that of the whole body—as opposed to details like the eyelids, lips or lashes—and since a healthy complexion requires a healthy body, the care of the complexion implies the care of the body. In the Pharaonic era, the body was first cleaned with water and natron to remove surface dirt and prepare the skin for the application of seven different perfumed oils from the ports of the Levant. For example, an unguent made of alabaster powder, natron and honey was used to firm the flesh; the use of a revitalizing oil, whose recipe was designed to "transform an old man into a young one," involved the following procedure: "Procure around two hectoliters of fresh fenugreek bulbs. Crush them. . . . When they are rubbed on the body, it becomes the perfect color. Baldness, freckles, age marks and all ruddiness are cured." The goal was already, according to the immortal phrase of Racine, to prevent or "repair years of irreparable insults." Ambroise Paré wrote about "special remedies that have the ability to disguise wrinkles and whiten the skin." He was referring to masks worn during the night and washed off in the morning.

The following era was to treat the problem of age in a singular manner. Time was obliterated: as soon as a child was born, it was made up. Said Diderot's *Encyclopédie:* "We are not content to use it [make-up] only when rosy cheeks have faded; we use it as early as childhood." Children were literally transformed into pint-sized old people; thanks to powder, everyone had white hair from the beginning to the end of his days. The generation gap disappeared in a cloud of white flour.

Following this interlude, beauty care products came back, with remedies that often did as much harm as good. An eighteenth-century ad for Eau de Ninon claimed that it would "preserve the perfect beauty, freshness and health of Ninon de Lenclos till the age of ninety." "L'Eau de Ninon contains calomel (mercurous chloride)," wrote Charles Girard, head of the municipal laboratory created in 1878 by the city's police department, in Marcellin Berthelot's *Grande Encyclopédie.* He continued: "Viard *veloutine* is composed of starch and zinc oxide. Common powders contain between thirty and ninety percent white lead. . . . Make-up products, through the metallic and toxic substances they contain, irritate and dry the skin by blocking the pores and preventing perspiration; they can cause serious illness."

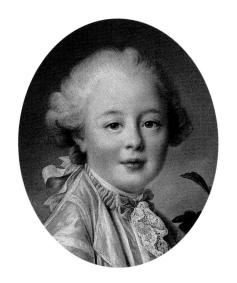

The Count of Nogent as a Child, detail, by François Hubert Drouais. Facing page: Caron advertisement from the 1950s.

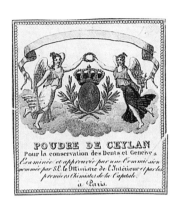

Cosmetic exoticism
from around 1830: Rouge from
the famous Piver house.
Facing page: A young woman
from the Empire period:
Self-portrait, by Constance
Mayer, detail, 1775–1821.

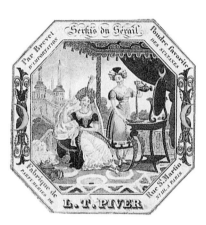

The recipe of Lola Montès, Countess of Lansfeld

"Take a small piece of benzoin gum and boil it in water until it forms a rich dye. Fifteen drops in a glass of water produces a mixture that resembles milk and releases a pleasant fragrance. It gives the cheeks a handsome pink color. If you let it dry on the face, it makes the skin clear and bright."

Concealing emotion

Education must precede the care of the body, since true beauty comes from the inside and shines through. The courtesan Lola Montès held the paradoxical belief that a woman is first of all a spiritual being. She interpreted the message of the fathers of the Church in her own way, by slightly laicizing the soul on the intellectual side of the word "spirit." "If it is true that the 'face is the mirror of the soul,' the recipe for a handsome face must be something that touches the soul. If a woman's soul is lacking in culture, taste and delicacy, if it doesn't have the joy of a happy spirit, all the mysteries of art will be impotent when it comes to giving her a beautiful face. This chaste, delightful activity of the soul, this spiritual energy that animates our bodies and lends them grace and shining light, is, after all, the true source of a woman's beauty. It gives eloquence to the language of her eyes; puts a smooth, pink hue on her cheeks; and lights up her entire person as if even her body were capable of thinking."

That's all very fine, but if we go too far back in the chain of cause and effect, we will end up at the flood, and make-up was not yet waterproof. In any case, a heavy coat of make-up, what might be called a glaze, not only blocks the

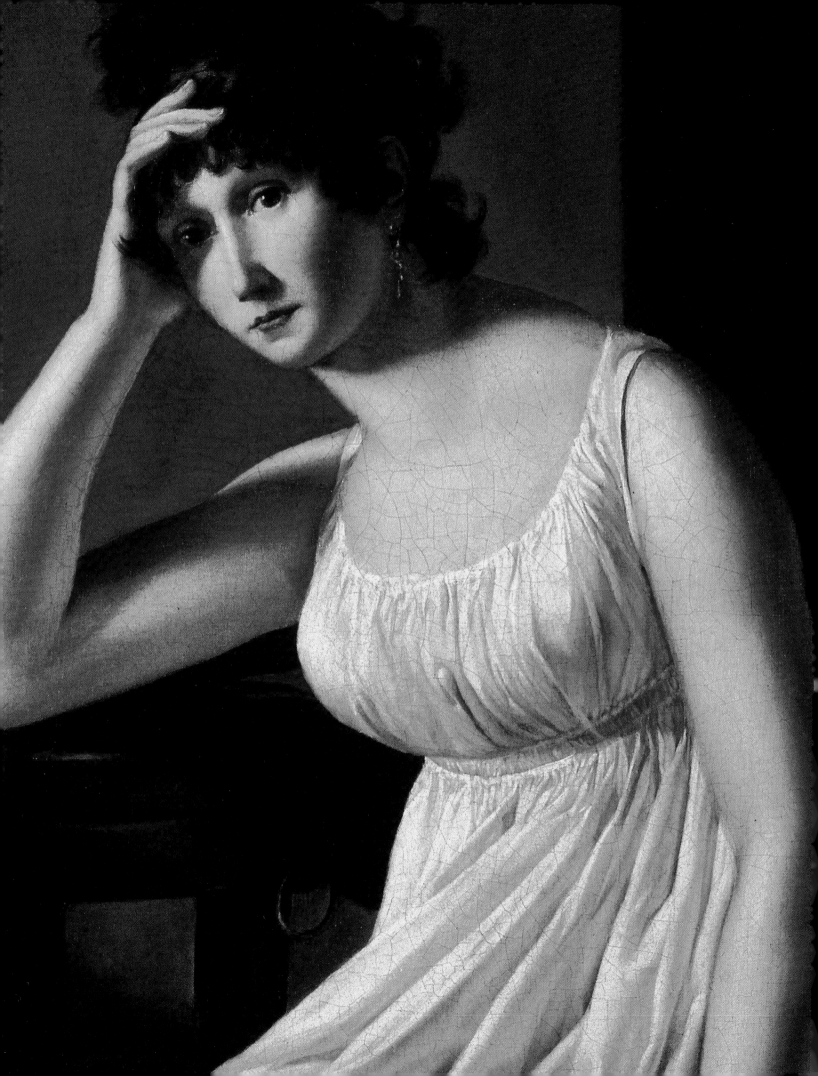

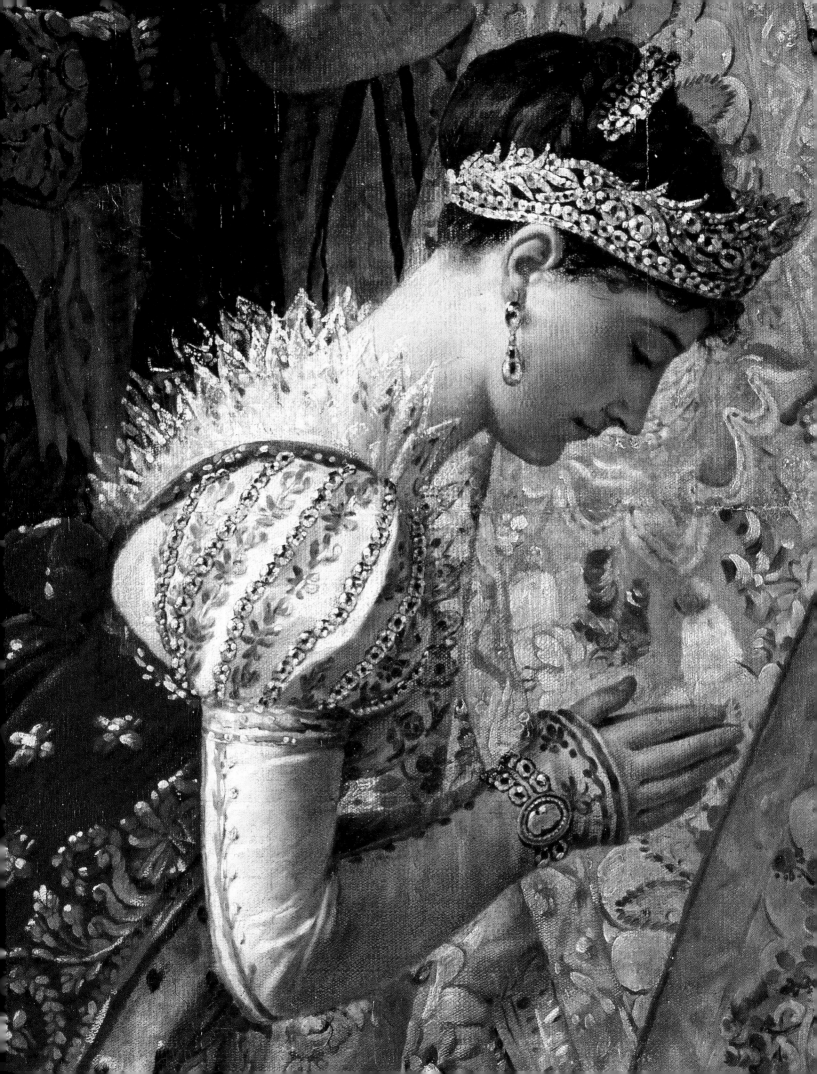

pores but also prevents any emotion from shining through—in fact, nothing shines through.

"The greatest charm of beauty lies in the expression," explained Miss Montès, who brought Louis de Bavière to his knees. But what expression can there be on a face "coated with paint and make-up? No blush of pleasure, no shiver of hope, no spark of love can shine on a plaster cast." If there is an expression, it is not, in the examples cited, the expression of oneself. In this case, what is being watched for—by the man, whose point of view Lola suddenly adopts—is not an expression but a reaction: the seducer observes what he has set off, what he inspires in his prey and how it responds.

When Lola was divulging her secrets, the era of uniform white complexions was coming to an end after a long run. When we read Ovid, we might be reading advertisements for detergents: "Come learn from me the art of turning your complexion a brilliant white." We are not, however, talking about scouring powder for the bathtub or sink but for the skin. "Every woman who coats her face with this cosmetic will make it more uniform, more brilliant than her mirror." A shiny nose is now about the most horrible thing that could happen to a woman, but there was a time when it was desirable to shine from the roots of the hair to the tip of the chin.

In the eighteenth century, there was no such thing as modulation: "The white of the forehead, more brilliant than in other places, darkens the slightest bit as it approaches the temples, where it seems slightly tinted with blue, while the outline of the lips should be as white as alabaster," was the advice of the *Bibliothèque des Dames*. In the second half of the following century, three new products were made available: Pink White for blonds; Yellow White, also known as Rachel White after the actress, for brunettes; and White White, for actors and eccentrics.

Empress Josephine's toilet kit, ordered from the cabinetmaker Félix Rémond in 1806, can be seen at Malmaison. It is mounted on a mahogany and burr elm pedestal table and contains crystal flacons; silver-gilt, tortoiseshell and porcelain boxes; and mother-of-pearl utensils. Each piece is marked with the initial "J."

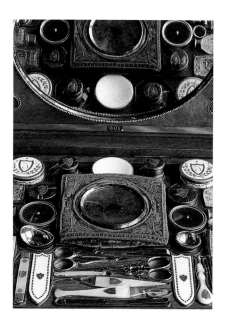

Facing page: *Coronation of Napoleon I and the Empress Josephine,* by Jacques Louis David, detail, 1805–07. Fearing that make-up would not sufficiently disguise the age difference between herself and Napoleon on the day of their coronation, Josephine asked J.-B. Isabey to paint her face.

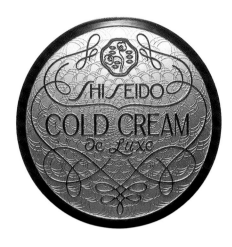

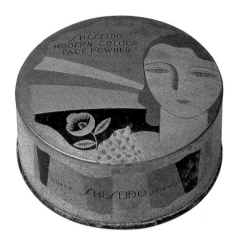

Left: The arabesque
and the camellia were the
symbols of the Shiseido
brand in 1932. Below:
An advertising photo taken
by François Kollar for l'Oréal
in 1930.

The many colors of white

At the end of the nineteenth
century, a matte finish replaced a
glossy one when rice powder—
really rice starch—was introduced.
Finer than wheat starch, it was
applied with a puff made of swan's
down, of which 420,000 were
produced each year in London
alone. The word "rice" didn't
necessarily mean anything either.
Everything imaginable could be
found in products sold under this
name, and they often contained
alabaster, which was heavier and
thus more profitable for the
merchant. "That explains why there
are a number of mills in La Villette
and Montmartre whose sole
purpose is to pulverize the alabaster
used by our perfumers."

Around 1920, powder existed
only in five shades, with three
fragrances. Elizabeth Arden had ten
shades for the cream used to fix the

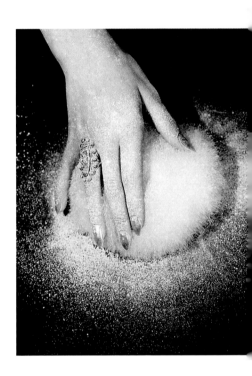

Facing page: A powder
puff as big as a swan.
Poster by Cappiello for
powder by Luzy, 1919.

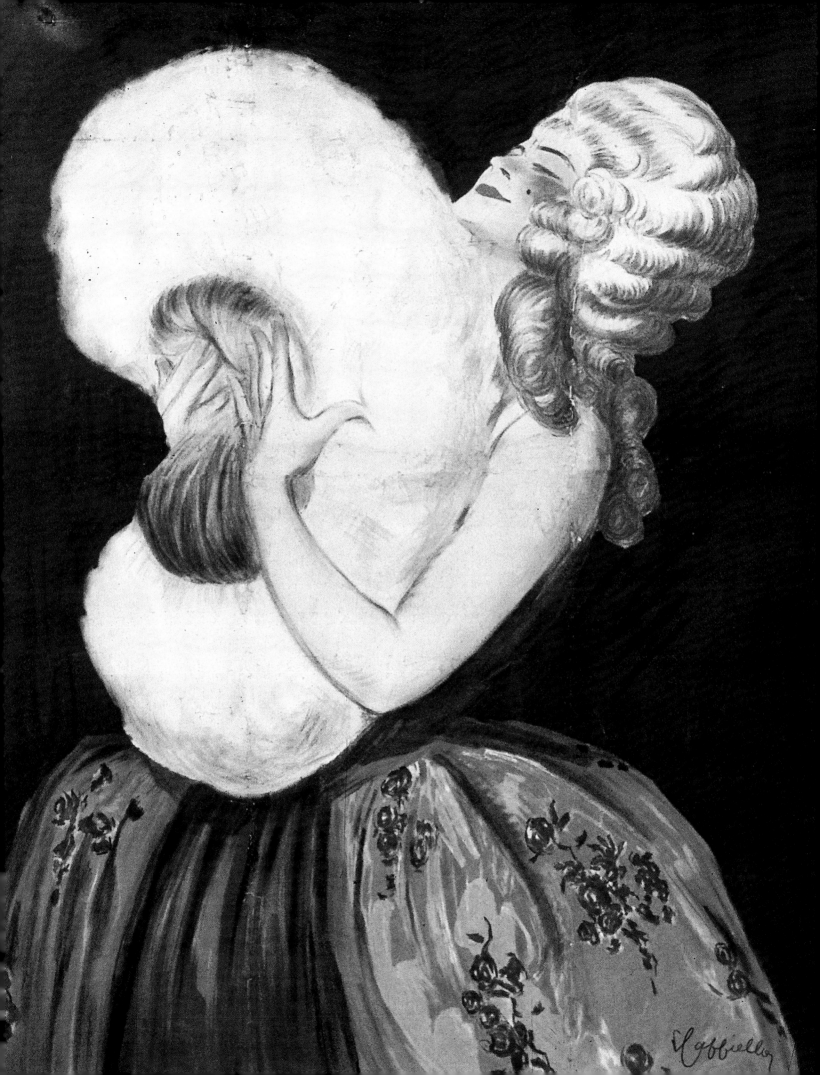

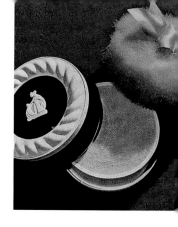

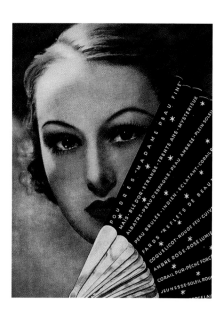

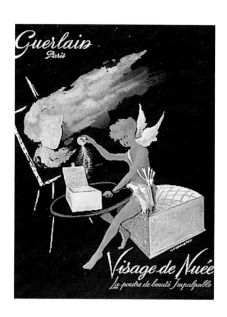

Caron's Grande Beauté
(left) and Guerlain's angel,
which now has arrows
and has become Cupid.

powder to the face, neck and hands, along with thirteen shades for Ardena Powder and six for Venetian Flowers Powder. Eighty years after she died, the actress who played Corneille and Racine's heroines remained the model for these palettes, with Rachel Pink, Special Rachel for light brown hair and Spanish Rachel for brunettes. Apricot was designated as "darker than Rachel" and designed especially for ivory complexions. Then there were light and dark shades of Rosetta for tanned complexions; Lily Powder, a mauve tone for evening; and green Almond, to lighten a highly colored complexion.

White powder was reserved for the neck and arms. The now wider palette of colors was used on the face. No more imitating statues—women were sculpting their own images.

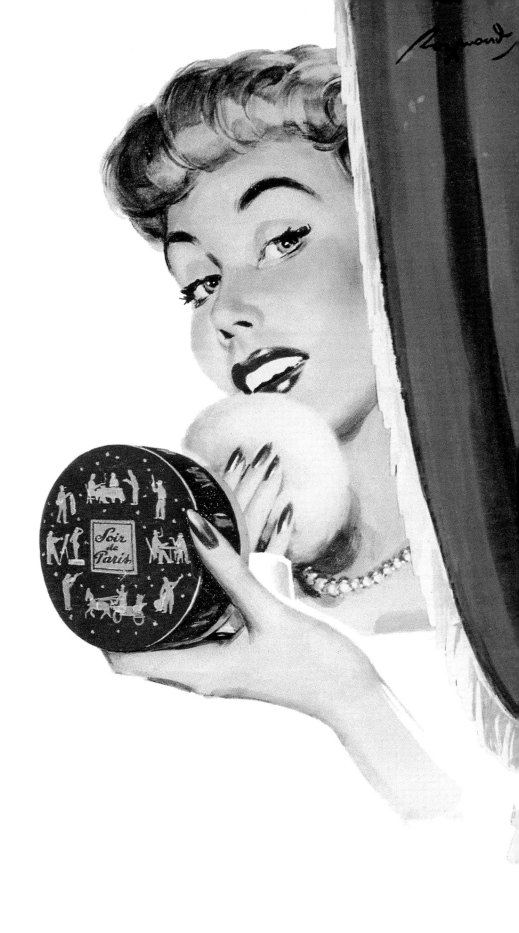

Baudelaire once paid homage
to a woman of (imitation) marble:
"Who doesn't understand that the
goal and result of using rice
powder—so inanely anathematized
by naive philosophers—is to erase
from the complexion all the outrages
that nature has left there and to
create an abstract unity in the grain
and color of the skin, a unity that . . .
immediately makes a human
resemble a statue, that is to say, a
divine, superior being?"

Helena Rubinstein addressed
herself to a woman of clay who
resculpts herself each morning with
her own hands. "Light colors add
relief, and dark ones have a slimming
effect, so you can model your face
by playing with shadow and light. In
no time at all, you will learn to use
foundations and powders of different
shades to create a new face for
yourself . . . and to show off what
you have to the best advantage."

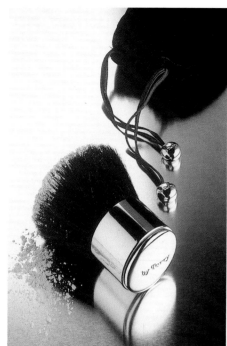

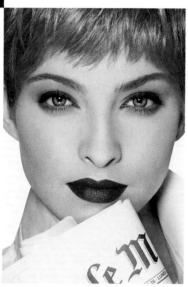

Diorever, spring 1999 (above) and Expressions du Regard, April 1996 (facing page): two looks created for Dior by Tyen, a photographer who takes his inspiration from painting and points out that Bacon based his paintings on photographs. Top left: Terry's loose powder.

Today's complexion

"Make the most of what you have." Make-up has become discreet: it does not emphasize its own qualities, but yours. Like those "flavor enhancers" that are added to food, it is there to serve you. This is a rather strange concept when you think about it: a woman buys a perfume for its own fragrance, not to enhance her body odor.

When Max Factor-Hollywood launched its Hi-Fi range of liquid make-ups in six shades, each corresponding to a complexion type, it claimed to be the "only one that does not change color after being applied to your skin" and promised to "make you ravishing without looking 'made up,' day and night. You will love its truly natural appearance; Hi-Fi softens and beautifies your face to perfection."

Soon a chart was created to compare ten shades of women's skin to seven shades of Hi-Fi, seven Creme Puff shades, eight pancake shades, seven cover-up sticks and eight powders. Meanwhile, Dior had created a range of fifteen shades that "reproduced" all complexions, from the lightest to the darkest. All new ranges were created in relation to these constants, which served as reference points for women.

Each product was presented differently, and the stages of the process became more diversified. To

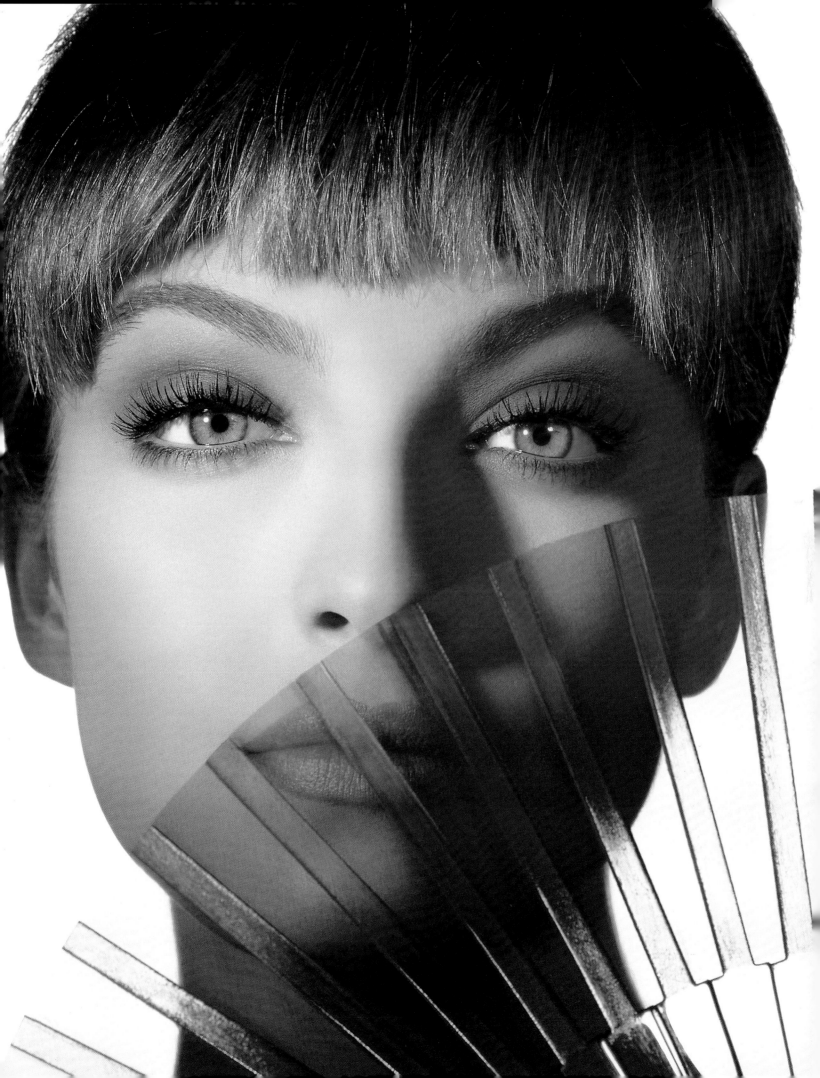

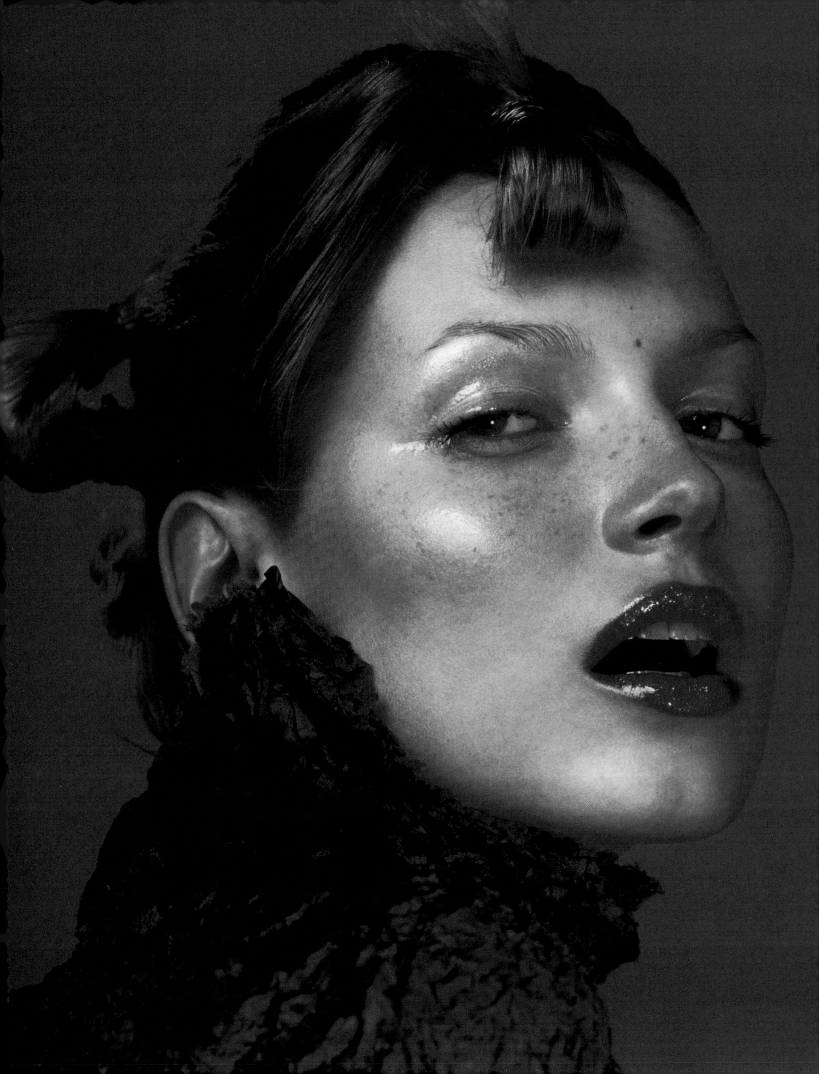

prepare the skin, women had to apply base cream, cover-up to hide imperfections and rings under the eyes, foundation to unify the complexion and loose powder to fix the foundation. The process became increasingly precise and technical: the gloss could now be found in the names. Forty years ago, Max Factor's Creme Puff products were already called Truly Fair, Tempting Touch, Twilight Blush, Candle Glow, Gay Whisper, Sun Frolic and Sun Goddess, plus the special Clair de Lune, which could be used for all complexions.

What is today's ideal complexion? A foundation is expected to make us "look healthy." It must be pinker or darker than the skin, which means we have to increase the amount of make-up on the face, as well as other visible areas, at the very least the neck. For several years now, European women (with the exception of the Italians, who still force themselves to do it) have dispensed with this chore by using on the face a foundation that is the same color as the neck. The idea is to unify the natural color of the skin and then add touches of color on the mouth and eyes. Pink has also more or less disappeared, except in the United States and the Middle East, where, for example, 718, a light, pinkish shade that was one of the first Dior foundations and has disappeared elsewhere, is still in demand.

Japanese women, who used to pinken their skin tone to appear more Western, have gone back to their natural complexions. Because their skin is thicker, the blood vessels are less apparent. They use light tones and neutral beige with a yellowish tint.

Overall, skin color has lightened up and become more luminous, while other facial colors are turning brown. After the heyday of matte finishes, we have come back to satiny, iridescent ones. The skin shines, and the reflections we so recently avoided are now gladly applied with the help of pearly pigments.

Preparations for a Lanvin fashion show in 1987. Cover-up is being applied to American model Sonia Cole.

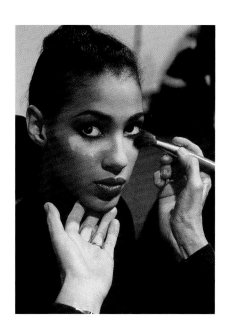

In the spring of 1999, Guerlain produced this compact containing Mozaïs eye shadow and Terracotta powder, for a "healthy look."
Facing page: A symphony in purple—Marta, cover girl of the December 1999 issue of *Zensé* magazine.

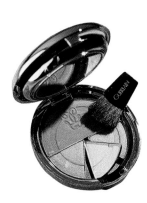

The eye

the window
to the soul

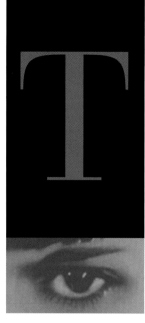

The eye is quite different from all the other parts of the body that can be made up. It is a two-way mirror: we look out at the world through the eye, and the world supposes that it can look into us the same way. In his *Éloge du maquillage,* Baudelaire describes the eye as a "window open onto the infinite": this could be taken as a rather prosaic description of the organ of sight which enables us to contemplate the stars . . . but it is unlikely that the poet intended such a simple interpretation, and we should no doubt look back through the "window," into the infinity of femininity.

The eye is the part of the human body where the soul shines through. Perhaps this is why eye make-up is the only kind of cosmetic mentioned in the Bible. In Racine's "adaptation" of a Biblical text, he included the face. "The borrowed brightness with which she carefully painted and adorned her face,"

writes Racine, whereas the Biblical version is simply: "She painted her eyes, adorned her head." In the Bible, even the receptacle for eye make-up is sanctified: after sending afflictions to test Job, God granted him a third daughter, who was christened *Keren-happuch,* ("horn of *pûk*"), referring to the recipient— originally a hollow horn—which contained the *pûk* used as eye-paint.

The product itself, which Indian Muslims use on the inner rim of the eyelids, is near-divine, according to the tradition of Jaffur Cherif's *Qanoûn-e-Islam,* quoted by Rimmel: "When God ordered Moses to show himself on Mount Sinai (Koh-e-Toor), the prophet fainted after glimpsing the heavenly countenance through a needle's eye. When he came to his senses, the mountain was on fire, and he made haste to go down; then the Sinai, addressing the Lord, cried: 'What! I am the smallest of your mountains and you have delivered me unto the flames!'

"The best recipe for bright eyes is not to go to bed late."
Lola Montès

Right: *Jeanne de Loynes,* by Amaury Duval, ca. 1860. Her gray eyes captivated Dumas fils. Jérôme Napoléon, the emperor's cousin, commissioned her portrait. Previous page: Katharine Hepburn in 1933.

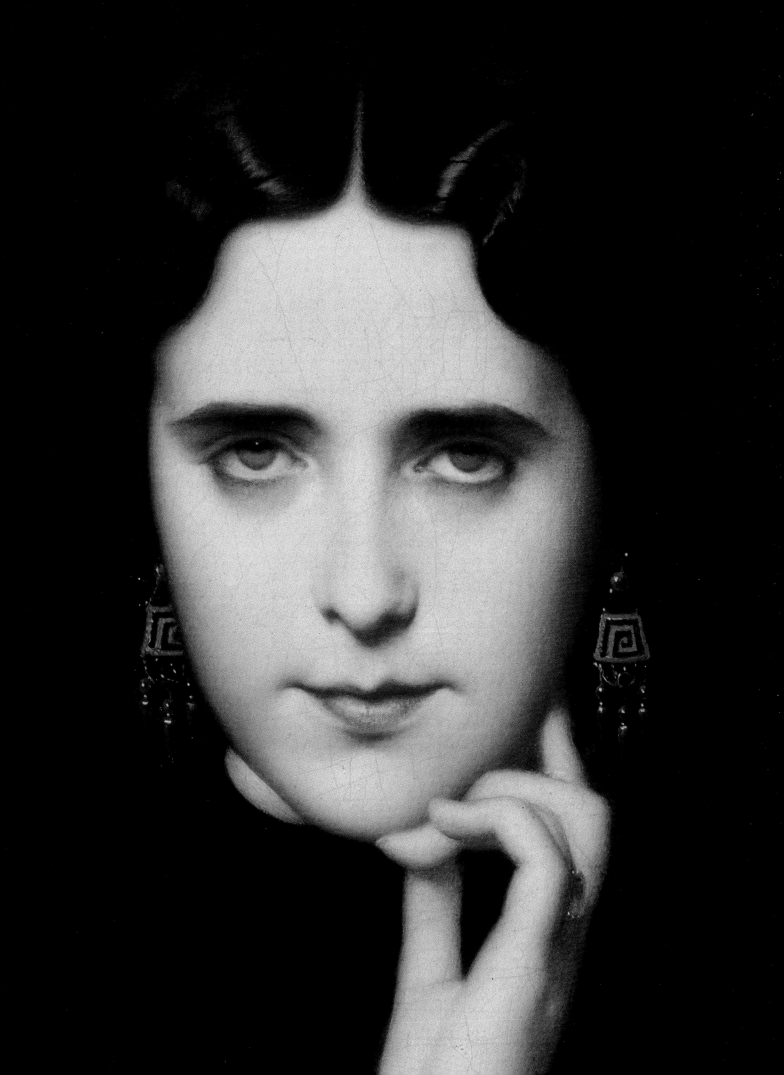

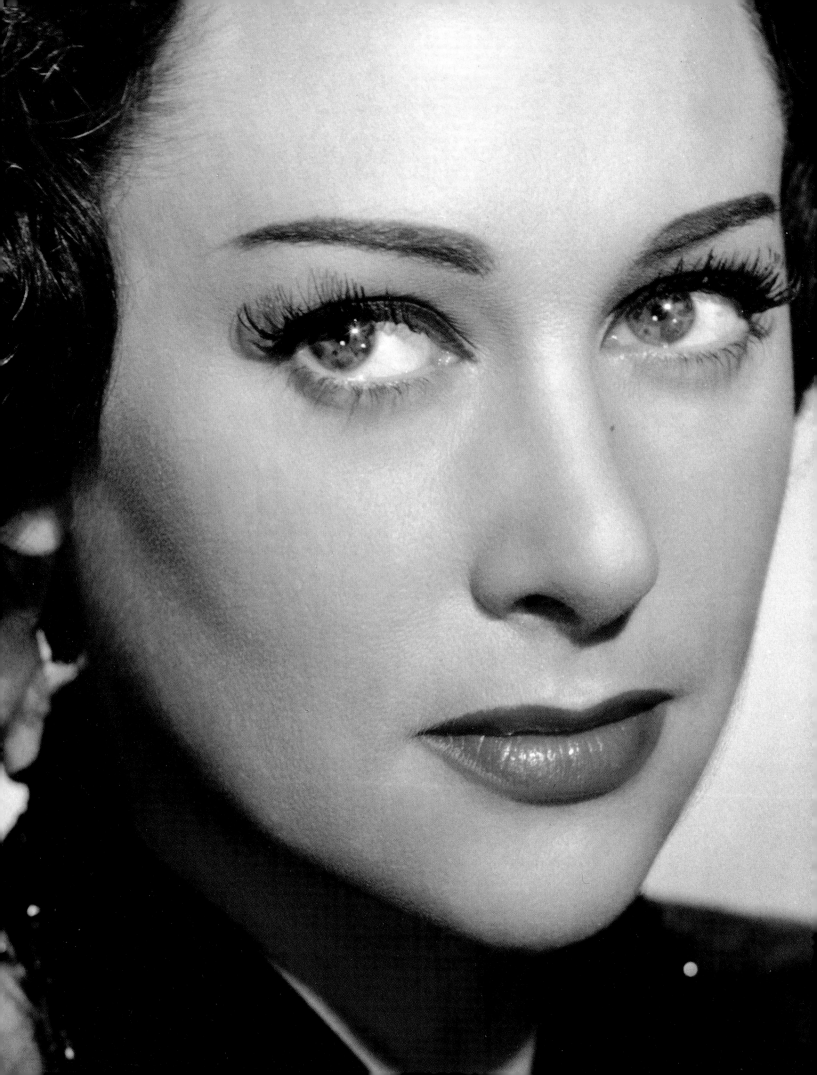

"So the Lord said to Moses: 'From this day on, you and your descendants shall reduce the earth of this mountain to powder, with which you shall rub your eyes.'" Ever since, Far Eastern Muslims have used *soûrma*—and that which is sold in Hindustani bazaars is supposed to be earth from Mount Sinai.

It would seem that Jewish women used make-up only on their eyes, Egyptian style. Antimony was used as well as kohl, which is still often the case in the Middle East. In translations of the Bible, "antimony" refers to the powdered antimony sulfide used on the eyes. The equivalent Greek word means "eye-enlarging."

Lingering looks

Since the dawn of civilization, wherever eyelashes have fluttered traces are to be found of the art of applying kohl—cases, corked bottles and sticks or stylets. Kohl is applied with a little wooden, ivory or silver stick, which tapers to a blunt end; the tip is moistened, sometimes with rose water, before being dipped in powder then used to draw a line along the inner rim of the eyelids. Lane tells us that the stick is called mirwed, *and the glass recipient in which the kohl is kept,* mukhula.

Excavations at Soleb, in Upper Nubia, unearthed a yellow earthenware kohl pot, with blue inscriptions naming the royal couple Amenophis III and Tiy (1403–1365 B.C.), and a glazed terracotta kohl case, decorated with flowers, with two tubes for sticks and spatulas. A box with three compartments indicates that there may have been three types of kohl for the three Egyptian seasons: the spring, the hot season, and the period when the Nile overflowed.

Museums exhibit black, olive-shaped Moroccan kohl bottles, encased in silver mesh, which date from the early nineteenth century. In Rimmel's book, there is a reproduction of a kohl case made of antelope skin, which was brought back to him from Africa (though he doesn't specify which region).

In the Deccan, it is traditional for a Muslim to give his fiancée a toilet bag, with a case containing soûrma, *which is used inside the eyelids, and* kajul, *to darken the eyebrows.*

Nowadays, the basic eye make-up kit includes an eyebrow pencil, a double eye shadow (one dark and one light), an eye pencil or liquid eyeliner to outline the eyes, and mascara for the eyelashes.

Double kohl case from Gezer, Israel, fourteenth century B.C.
Left: A triple row of eyelashes for Martine Carol in the Max Ophuls film *Lola Montès*, 1957.

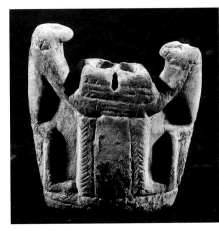

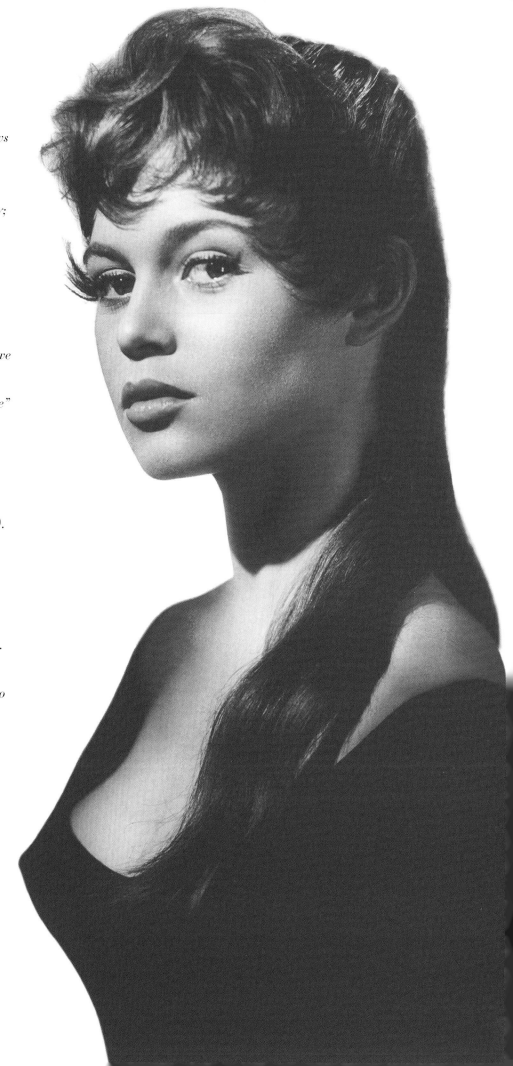

"*Black. Black eyes are greatly admired,
and women who are lucky enough to have
them, with a white complexion,
take care to darken their hair and eyebrows
to add to the dramatic effect.*

*Eyebrows. Finely arched eyebrows are
one of the thirty-six prerequisites of beauty;
d'Alix knows this, and paints them black,
to attract attention to them.*

*Eyes. For little maidens, to have pretty
eyes is almost a guarantee of fortune.
When they are lucky enough to own such
a pair, they take pains to practice expressive
looks in the mirror, using their eyes to
win hearts and receive applause and praise*"
(*Caraccioli*, Dictionary).

"*As the eye reflects the soul,
and as worthy souls are few, beautiful
eyes are few and far between*"
(*Louis Sébastien Mercier*, Tableau de Paris).

"*HER. A thin girl, alone in a bedroom,
sitting or half-lying on a crumpled bed.
The bedroom's untidy, hasn't been aired
for ages. Neither has the girl, but she's
wearing make-up, old mascara at any rate.
She looks like a student who went to bed
without taking off her make-up, like they do
sometimes, and who's just woken up.*"
(*J. Serena*, Rimmel).

Bigger, brighter, and more beautiful

Eye make-up tries to do three things: firstly, to make the eye bigger—to open the window wider onto the unfathomable mystery of the soul; secondly, it aims to make the eye brighter, to add to its sparkle; thirdly, it is used to decorate lashes and brows—though the meaning of this painting is open to interpretation.

Théophile Gautier sums up this triple aspect in a single sentence: "Eye-paint is much disapproved: but those painted lines lengthen the eyelids, define the curve of the eyebrows and bring out the brilliance of the eyes, like the finishing touches that a painter might give to a masterpiece."

The trilogy ("enlarging, brightening, decorating") is a recurrent theme. According to Haafner, "Indian bayaderes paint the rims of their eyelids black with *tschokko tschaâi,* a mixture of which the main ingredient is antimony. This paint makes their eyes look very bright, and bigger than they really are."

In the Arab world at the end of the first millennium, the eyebrows were painted with a decoction of *wasma,* a sort of indigo; the eyes were enlarged with Ispahan kohl, applied with a little ivory stick.

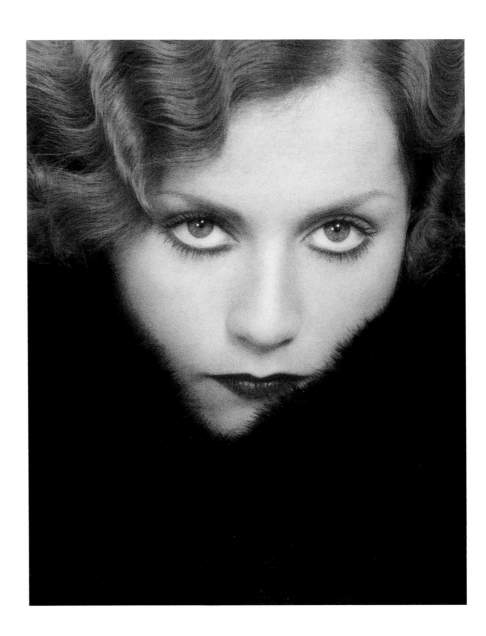

The pallid complexion and intense gaze of the femme fatale: Isabelle Huppert in the Claude Chabrol film *Violette Nozière,* 1976. Left: Tousled hair and long lashes—Brigitte Bardot in 1954, aged twenty. She had already appeared in *La Fille sans voile* and *Le Portrait de son père.*

"The Shiseido eye."
Advertisement for the
solid perfume May, 1978.

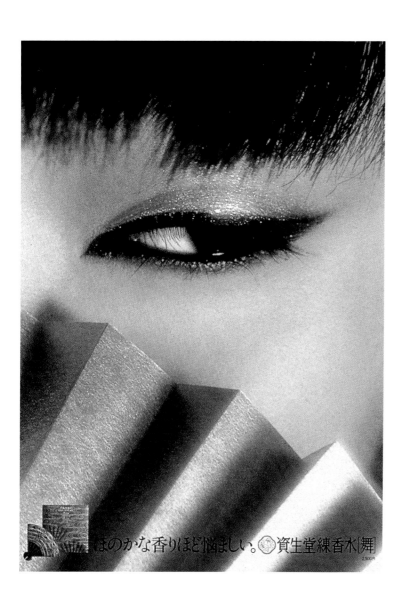

ほのかな香りほど悩ましい。◎資生堂練香水[舞]

Roman women used to make
their eyes look bigger by drawing a
dark line under them with fuligo, a
lampblack obtained from various
fatty, aromatic substances. In
Byzantium, it was fashionable to
have thin eyebrows, dyed black,
and black eyes enlarged with kohl
made from the incomplete
carbonization of various fatty plants.
Tertullian denounced this "blackish
powder used to color and lengthen
the eyelids."

Eye make-up intended to make
the eye look larger is fairly clear-cut,
but eyebrow-painting is open to
interpretation. In China, the fashion
which consisted of shaving the
eyebrows off to paint new ones on
in blue or black ink lasted for
twelve centuries—if that can still be
called a fashion! In the first century
B.C., they were painted in the
shape of upturned "V"s, and in
the first century A.D. they became
curves that extended halfway up
the forehead.

Right: Kohl stylet, eyelash
curlers, eyeliner brushes:
eye make-up accessories
always seem particularly
aggressive . . . as if
reminiscent of the
punishment inflicted on
Oedipus for his
transgression. Advertising
visual, 1955.

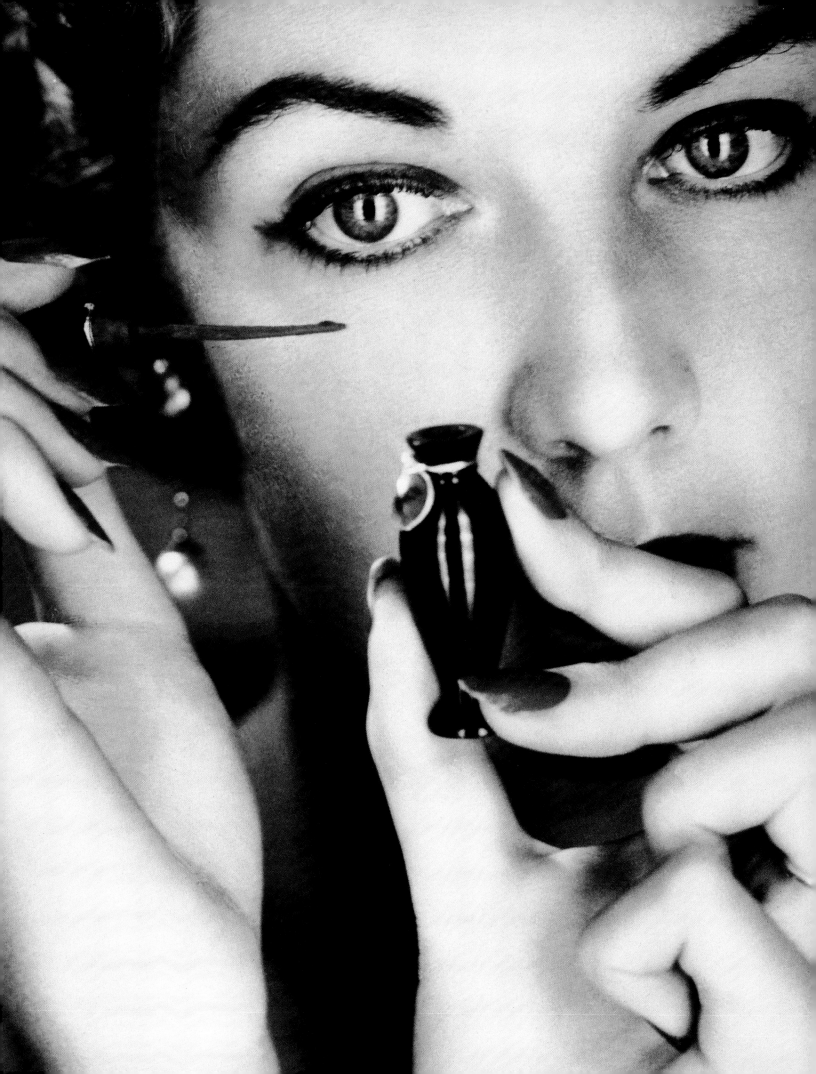

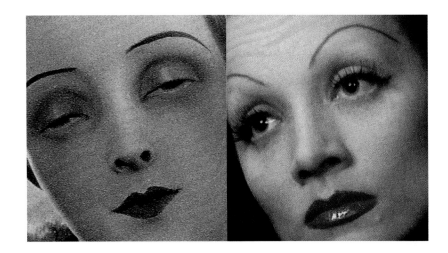

1930s: Heavy eyelids under plucked, arching eyebrows— Siegel's still life next to the tragic expression of Marlene Dietrich . . .
During the Renaissance, it was customary to "peel" ones eyebrows, perhaps in an attempt to resemble the rediscovered statues of Antiquity.
Right: A Young Lady, by Petrus Christus (ca. 1470).

Careful calligraphers

Renaissance ladies shaved off not only their eyebrows, but also their hair, from the hairline almost up to the top of their heads; perhaps this was an attempt to correspond to the ideal of beauty represented by the rediscovered sculptures of classical Antiquity. In nineteenth-century Japan, however, shaved eyebrows, like blackened teeth, were the distinguishing feature of the married woman.

Flaubert, always a reliable source of information, tells us that in Carthage, Salammbô's nurse "lengthened her eyebrows with a mixture of gum, musk, ebony and crushed flies' legs." Doctor James, with all the authority of a medical man, tells us that fifteenth-century Russian ladies (like Martial's Roman women) wore false eyebrows.

In the early nineteenth century, Caron (who inspired Balzac's César Birotteau) explained that "in France, a beautiful eyebrow must be arched and very fine, with lustrous black hairs." And at the end of the same century, James maintained that, whatever the preferences regarding color, there was still one golden rule: the arch!

"We also require them to be well separated," added Caron. This was already the case in the Middle Ages and during the Renaissance, when eyebrows had to be "well-ordered, thin and very fine like a little brushstroke," and above all "set well apart."

On the other hand, in Buddhist paintings from the Ajanta caves, the eyebrows meet above the nose: we know that this double curve reproduced the shape of the archer's

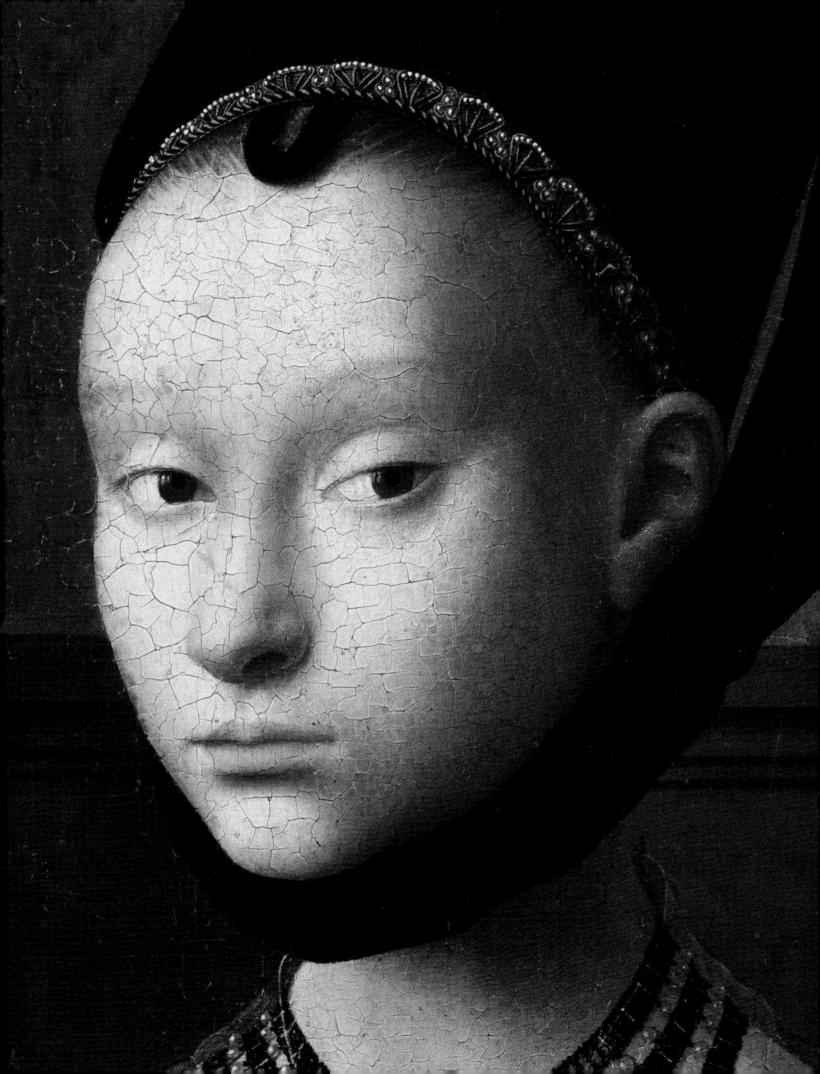

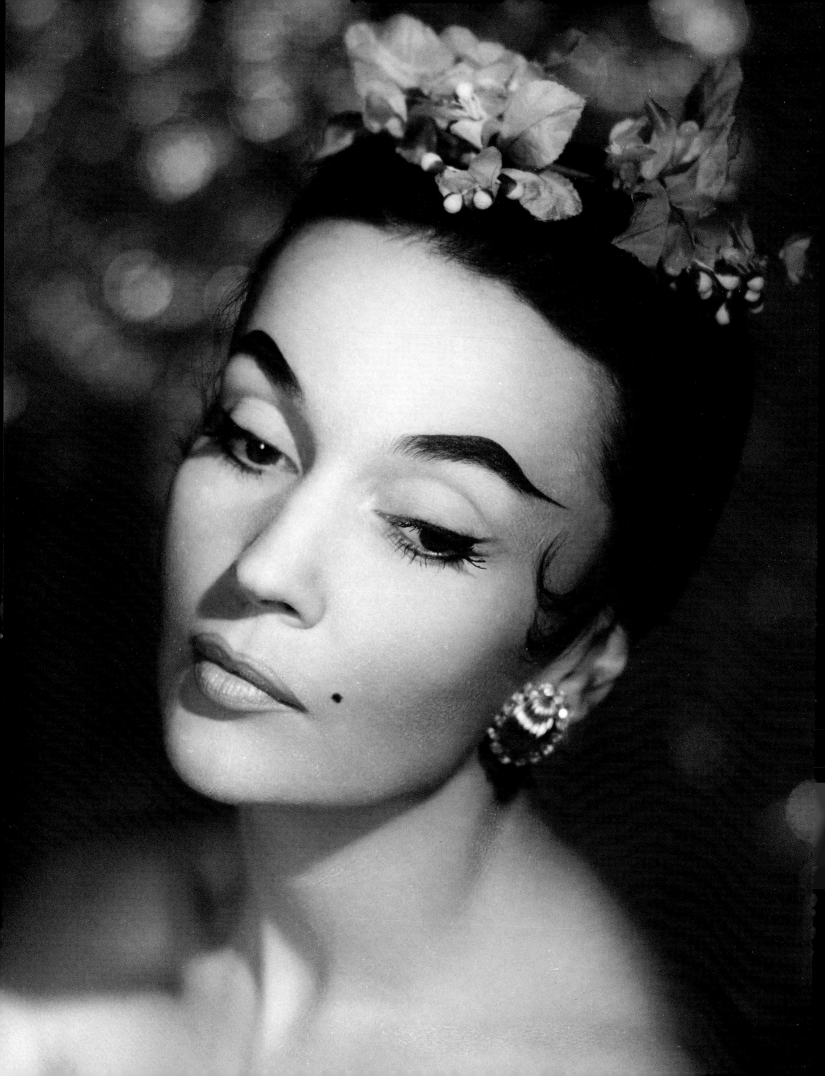

bow, in an art form which did not concern itself primarily with realism. Eliane Gouriou, Dior's international make-up consultant, takes a psychological approach to make-up: "It is first and foremost a language. Louise Brooks' eyebrows, for example, in *Pandora's Box*, are drawn very low, and go right down to the inner corner of her eyes. This gives her a sad, indeed a tragic look, which together with her black-rimmed eyes seems to say: 'I keep my distance from the world, I internalize my emotions, I observe, and this gives me greater depth and strength.' Marlene Dietrich's eyebrows, however, are rounded, well apart, long and very high above her eyes, thereby saying: 'I am open to the world, I leave room for sensitivity, fantasy and imagination.'"

Louise Brooks on the cover of *Motion Picture Classic*. Her short eyebrows are like the stylized wings of an airline-company logo. Left: Ludmilla Tcherina, star of the Monte-Carlo ballet, with soaring eyebrows, 1957.

Hair-removing horrors

"To remove the hairs which disadvantage the eyebrows," according to Alexis, in The Secrets of Lord Alexis: recipes from various authors, *1691, "you must carefully pluck and pull out the unsightly hairs of the eyes; then anoint the place with warm goat's blood, or the blood of a hare or a bat, or else you must rub it with the milk of a she-dog, or with a copper needle, which has been much heated and cooled in vinegar; touch the place with it, and the hairs will not reappear.*

To keep the plucked hairs from returning to the eyes, you must burn leeches in an earthen pot; reduce them to ashes, and apply these to the place whence the hairs have been plucked: they will not grow back."

Lane tells us that bat's blood was also used in nineteenth-century Egypt, where it was applied as a depilatory or to prevent hair-growth in newborn baby girls.

elle a les yeux Dior...

Waterproof make-up for
a mermaid's eyes:
Dior eyeshadow, by
Gruau, 1971.
Right: One of Baron de
Meyer's last fashion
photographs for *Harper's
Bazaar* in 1931. The models
chosen by the famous baron
became increasingly ethereal
and stylized, and were
eventually replaced by
window-dummies.

Passion . . . or fashion?

Eyebrow painting may require
interpretation, but bright eyes appear
to tell their own story. The eye is a
mirror that reflects colors applied
nearby (in the corners, on the
eyelids, or even on the cheeks); but
it also reflects the emotions . . . and
maybe the colors are sometimes
applied to feign sentiment!

"Paint your eyes with the humble
modesty that comes from a well-
ordered mind"; this was the only
kind of "make-up" that Tertullian
would accept. "The eyes have been
called the 'windows of the soul',"
wrote Lola Montès, "and this only
goes to reinforce . . . everything
I have said about the influence of
passion on beauty." Whether the
eye shines with humble modesty
or devouring passion, it hardly

matters: in both cases it reflects
natural feelings.

The Indian poet Kalidasa looked
to nature for the expression of
beauty: his messenger-cloud
compares the eyes of the beloved to
those of the timid gazelle, and finds
"the wave of her eyebrows in the
gentle ripple of the stream."

Nature sometimes needs a
helping hand, however, and a touch
of rouge near the eye can produce
the same effect as an authentic
passion. To give their eyes extra
brightness, Greek women used to
color their lower lids with a flesh-
colored shadow tinged slightly pink,
made from a blend of red and yellow
ochers, and perhaps white earth. In
Ovid's *Ars Amatoria,* he says: "You
are not ashamed to add sparkle to
your eyes with a fine ash (charcoal,

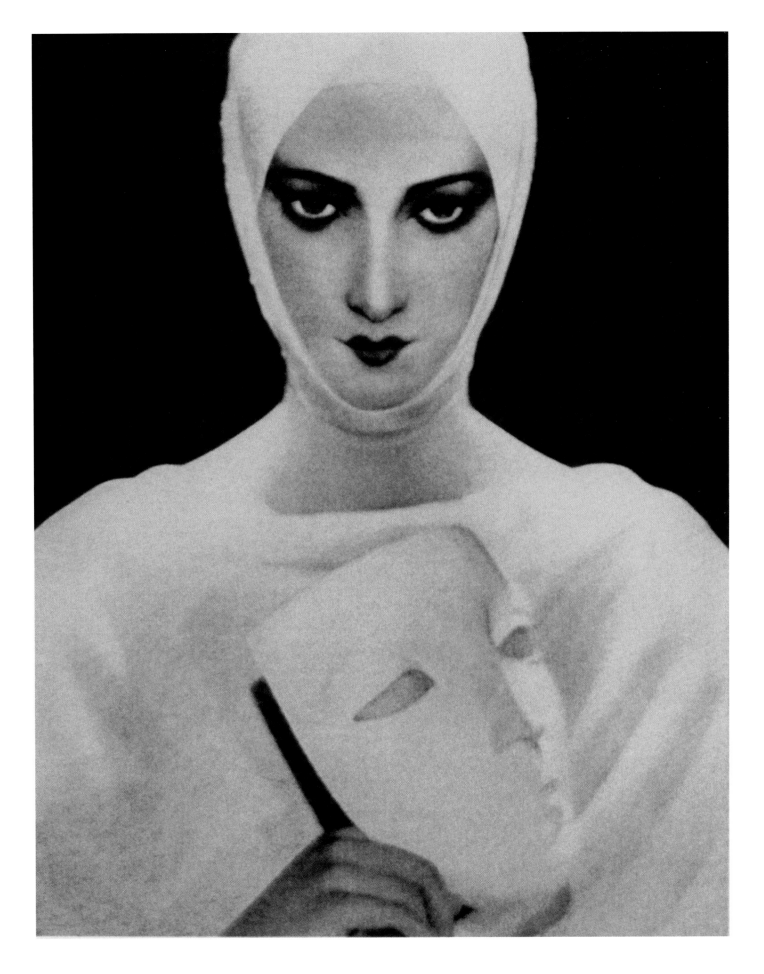

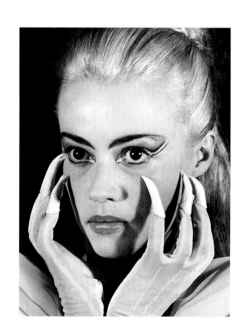

Jeanne Moreau in
Jean Cocteau's *La Machine
infernale*, 1954: eyelashes
and eyebrows meet in a
dramatic sweep.

or burnt rose petals), or with the saffron that grows on the banks of the Cydnus." James, who lived at a time when women used little eye make-up, considered that the eyelids could be darkened a natural, tawny color, evoking the complexion of Andalusian women and hinting at southern passion. This kind of make-up was common in the theater: in *The Dancer*, a print by Kunisada, we see a *kamuro* applying rouge to the corner of her eyes. In close-ups from the film *The Red Shoes*, the red discs that Moira Shearer had on each side of her nose, near her eyes, are clearly visible.

With make-up, one can bring inner feelings to the surface and express them in color: the red glow of a cheek puts fire in the eyes. The theater teaches a twofold lesson: how to feign an emotion, and how to portray it through make-up.

According to Laclos, "We are well aware that the great passions of the soul or the senses are reflected in the eyes, even when obstacles are put in their way. Nature has it so; and art has sought to imitate nature, with some success. This use of artifice can often be seen in the theater, but its misuse is increasingly common in society: appearances have become deceptive, and eyes are no longer to be trusted. Cosmetics assist this perfidy; according to travelers' reports, the bayaderes of Hindustan use a powder which enables them to wear an expression of pleasure, but keep their eyes brimming over with warm, voluptuous tears (according to Lola Montès, Spanish women used orange juice for the same purpose); and European women apply rouge to their cheeks to make their eyes shine with ardent desire."

Blood red was the prerogative of the vamp, who conquered the silver screen with a sweep of her dark lashes.

Right: Moira Shearer and
Robert Helpmann in the
film-ballet *The Red Shoes,* 1948.
Powell and Pressburger then
made *The Tales of Hoffmann,*
each was treated in a different
color: ocher for Olympia,
purple for Giuletta, and indigo
for Antonia.

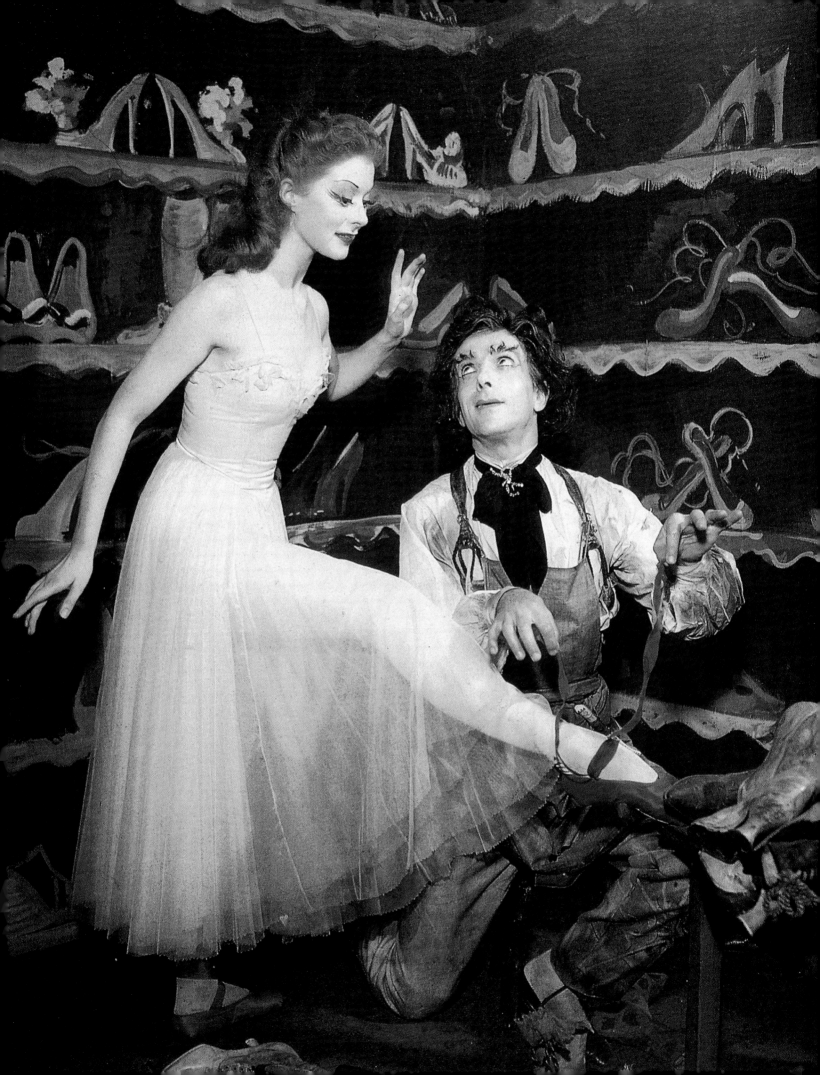

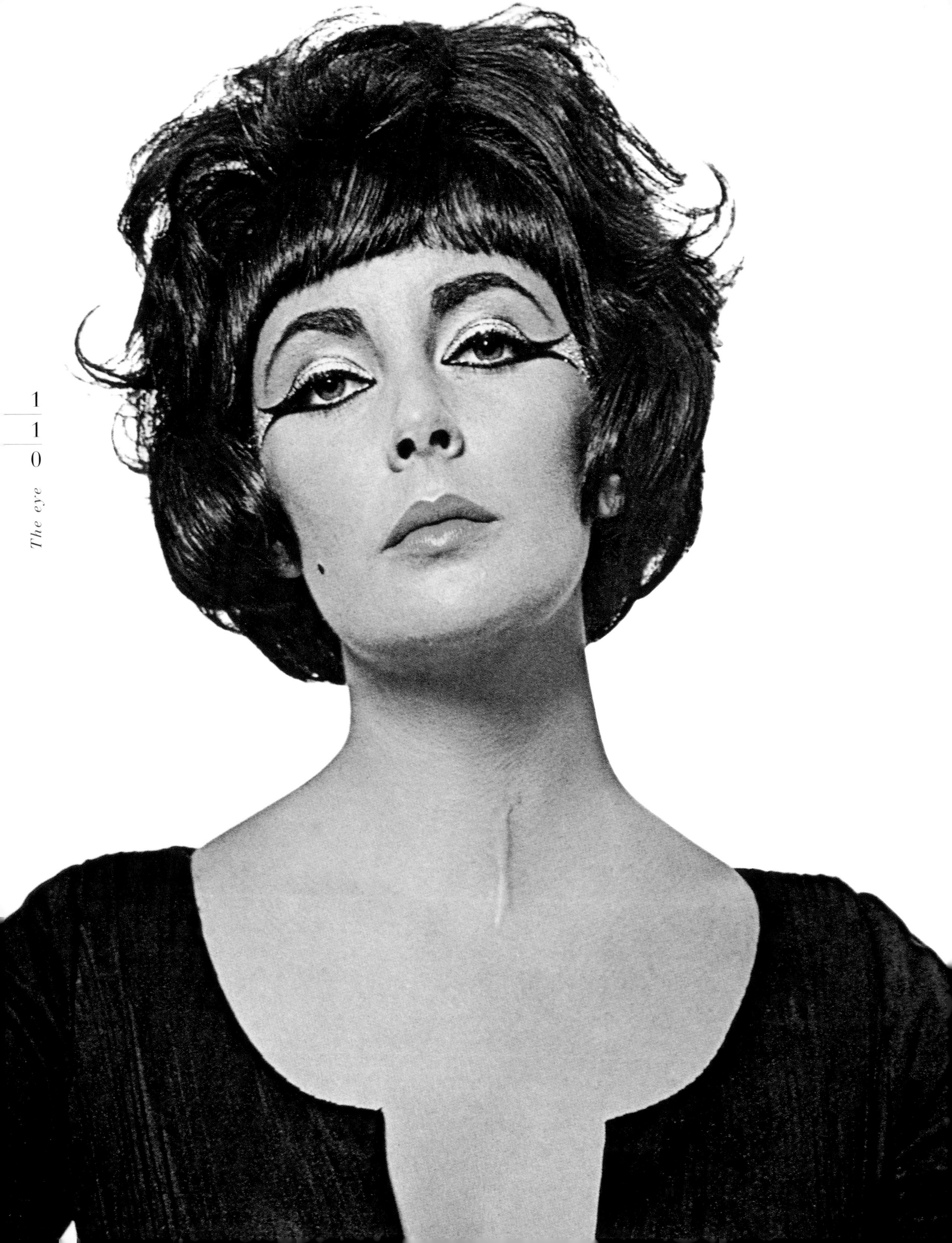

"Theda Bara, the 'siren of the silent movie' (she played Sappho, Carmen, Salome, Cleopatra, Madame du Barry . . .) became world-famous for her vampish look, which was created by our make-up," wrote Helena Rubenstein. "Nobody in America made up their eyes. In France, a few theater actresses used mascara . . . but the result was not always very successful. So I created a mascara for Theda Bara that made the most of her wonderfully expressive eyes, so that they became the focal point of all attention. What's more, the mascara didn't run! Finally, I added a touch of shadow to her eyelids. The result was extraordinary! All the papers and magazines reported the event—but Theda Bara made an even greater sensation the day she painted her toenails for the first time!"

Shadows of the past . . .

Thousands of years before the vamp, there was the scribe. Eye make-up is so old that it can be used as a means of dating: green make-up around (male or female) Egyptian eyes dates from around 2700 B.C.; black make-up is from a later period. The famous painted limestone statue of a seated scribe has green make-up around the eyes, and dates from a period between 2620 and 2350 B.C.

The earliest known form of eye shadow was a malachite powder (natural copper carbonate, of a lovely mottled green color), then, from the Third Dynasty onward, the fashion

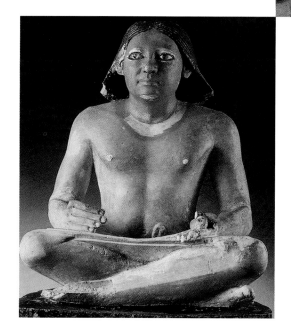

Seated scribe from the early fifth dynasty, ca. 2500 B.C., and detail from a mummy's mask. Left: Elizabeth Taylor in 1974. Eleven years after Cleopatra she still had Egyptian eyes! Mishima remembers the character's "melancholy eyes, with heavily painted lids."

Masculinity and mascara

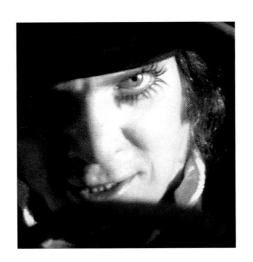

When writer Pierre Loti was about to leave for Morocco with the French ambassador (who was to present his credentials to the sultan), he noted: "March 20, 1889. I have suppressed the rouge that I used to insist on wearing on my cheeks; it made me look old and gaunt. (He was thirty-nine at the time.) My unpainted face is more distinguished and younger-looking, and my eyes look finer against this pallor. In Morocco, I shall enlarge them a little again, in the Arab fashion. This will be my desert vanity . . ."

"Aschenbach sat back indolently, incapable of resisting; indeed he was filled with new hope at the sight he saw in the mirror, as his eyebrows acquired a smooth, elegant arch, and his eyes began to slant, bigger and brighter thanks to a touch of kohl beneath the lids . . . 'The Signore may now fall in love without fear'," says the hairdresser in Thomas Mann's Death in Venice.

Two legendary figures from the 1970s: Malcolm McDowell in Stanley Kubrick's *A Clockwork Orange,* 1971 (above), and Mick Jagger in *Performance*, a film by Nicholas Roeg and Donald Cammel, 1970 (opposite). Eyelashes no longer create a languid, doe-eyed look; they have turned into the hairy legs of predatory insects.

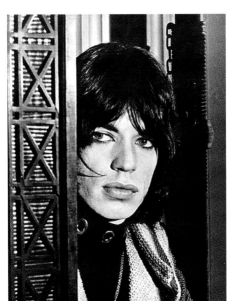

Everyone remembers Malcolm McDowell's made-up eye when he played Alex, the young gang-leader in A Clockwork Orange. The film was made in 1971, and mascara was becoming a symbol of virility, like a pirate's or gypsy's earring. David Bowie was a master in the art of make-up, and in fact almost all rock stars, from Mick Jagger and Keith Richard to Jacques Higelin, have worn eye make-up at some stage in their career.

was for kohl or antimony, which, in the form of sulfur, was plentiful on the eastern banks of the Red Sea; it was applied with a stylus, to outline and enlarge the eyes.

In Greece, eye make-up was always dark-colored (as it became in Egypt). There were two products, called *stimmis* and *asbolê*, with which specialized chambermaids used to paint the rim of the eyelids at the root of the lashes, the lashes themselves and the eyebrows. *Stimmis* was a bright black or bluish color; it was composed of antimony (silvery powdered sulfur), and galenite (natural lead sulfide of a dazzling bluish-gray, which was plentiful on the islands of the Aegean Sea and in Asia Minor, and was originally used to paint vases), with bismuth as an excipient. *Asbolê* was a matte lampblack, a soot resulting from the combustion of pine leaves,

wet pitch, aromatic resins, oleaginous plants and almond shells, which was fixed with a mixture of egg-white and gum ammoniac.

Eye make-up was here to stay, and nothing changed for a long time. Gallic ladies simply added an ingredient to the soot, to paint their eyebrows: a liquid extracted from the garfish, an elongated fish with long toothed jaws that was fished near the coast. In the Middle Ages, the eyelids were given special treatment: "The skin under a woman's eye sometimes becomes discolored and livid," said Ruelle, who suggested the following remedy: "Let the woman bathe her face in warm water, and rub well with a finger on the discolored part. Then take some wheat, rub it in well, and wipe with a cloth. Repeat several times, and the treated area will acquire a fine color."

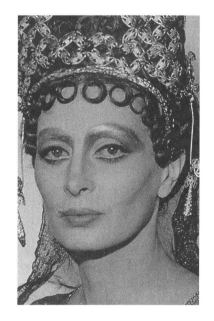

Capucine's extravagant baroque make-up in *Fellini's Satyricon*, 1969.

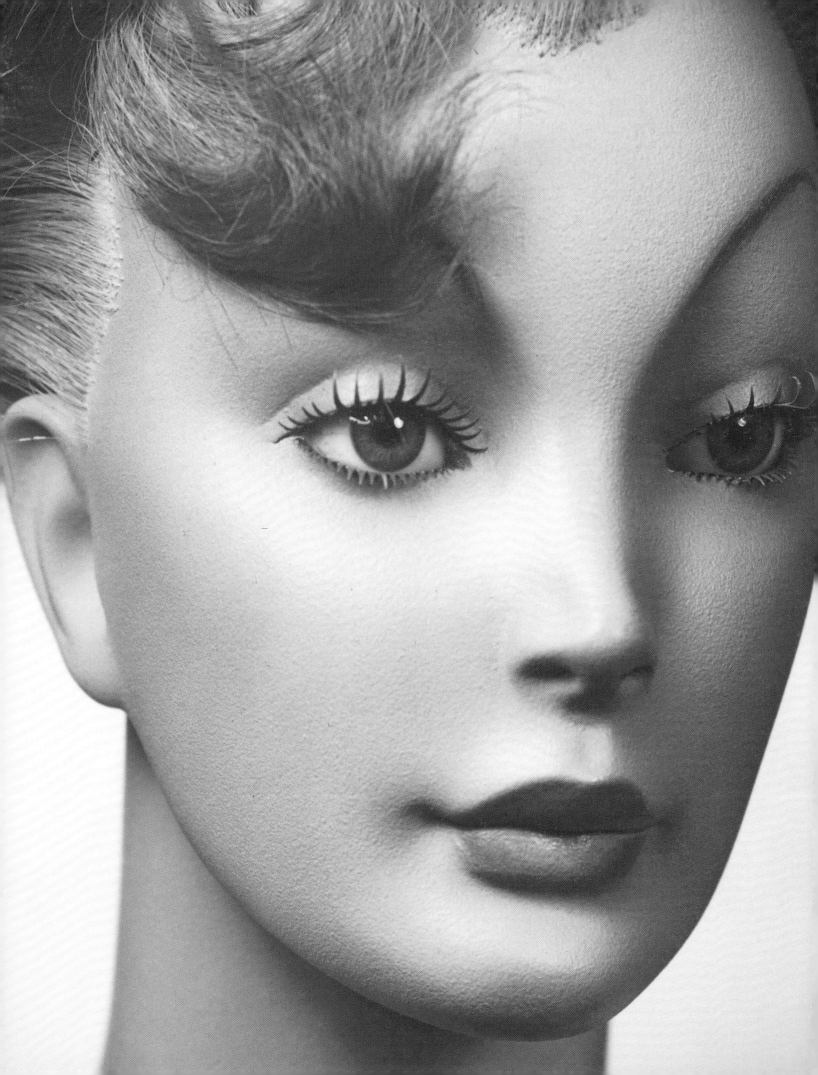

Lashing out...

In the nineteenth century, in the suburbs of Cairo, Lane reports that he twice saw perfect reproductions of Pharaonic make-up. The use of kohl was "a universal practice among women of the upper and middle classes, and very common in the lower classes; they make their kohl with a lampblack produced by burning almonds or an incense of ordinary quality called *liban*. There are many others sorts, composed of the powder of various lead ores, to which they often add sarcocolla, pepper, sugar candy, the fine powder of a Venetian sequin and sometimes pearls reduced to powder. Antimony is said to have been used in the past."

The Jewish women of Tunis and Tangiers used Egyptian kohl to create their gentle doe-eyed look, according to Eugène Rimmel— member and reporter of the international jury at the World Fair in 1862, and assistant commissioner at that of 1867. Here is the recipe given him by one of his correspondents, Mr. A. Chapelié of Tunis, which he guaranteed to be genuine: "A mixture of *alquifou* (lead sulfide) and burnt copper is put into a lemon, which is then placed on the

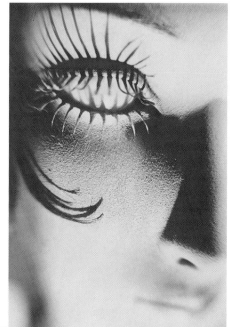

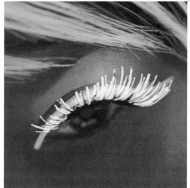

Eyelashes made up one by one, by J.-H. Lartigue (above), and by Tyen (left): a bright plumage, for a tropical background. Below: Mascara by Lancôme.
Facing page: Italian mannequin for Rosa, ca. 1935. "Write to Mlle du Gué and ask her to send you the doll that Mme de Coulanges sent her. Then you will see how to do this (hairstyle)."
Mme de Sévigné, May 6, 1671.

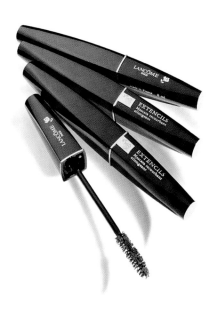

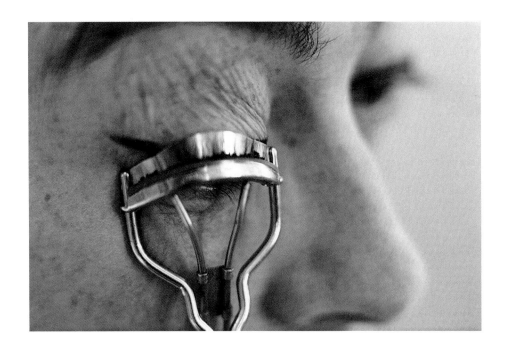

Joan Crawford curling her eyelashes: this efficient beauty aid looks like an instrument of torture! It was widely used, however, in the days before "long lash" mascara.
Right: A make-up scene in Tokyo in the 1980s.

fire; when the whole thing is sufficiently carbonized, it is crushed with coral, sandalwood, fine pearls, amber, a bat's wing and a piece of chameleon. This mixture is then burnt again, reduced to a fine powder and sprinkled with scented water."

A Ming engraving from the fifteenth century shows one of the favorite wives of Yang-ti (whose reign began in 604) painting her eyebrows, holding a circular mirror in her left hand. According to James, nineteenth-century Western beauties made up their eyes to create an oriental, almond-shaped look, "à la Chinoise."

The eyes may have been the first feature to be made up, but human inventiveness in the art of beautification knows no bounds, and contemporary make-up can still contribute something new. Chinese and Japanese women did not make up their eyelashes, which were very short. The women in European paintings from the sixteenth and seventeenth centuries, far from making up their eyelashes, often have none at all. For a long time, nobody seems to have paid much attention to the length of the eyelashes, but they were to become an important feature in a woman's appearance.

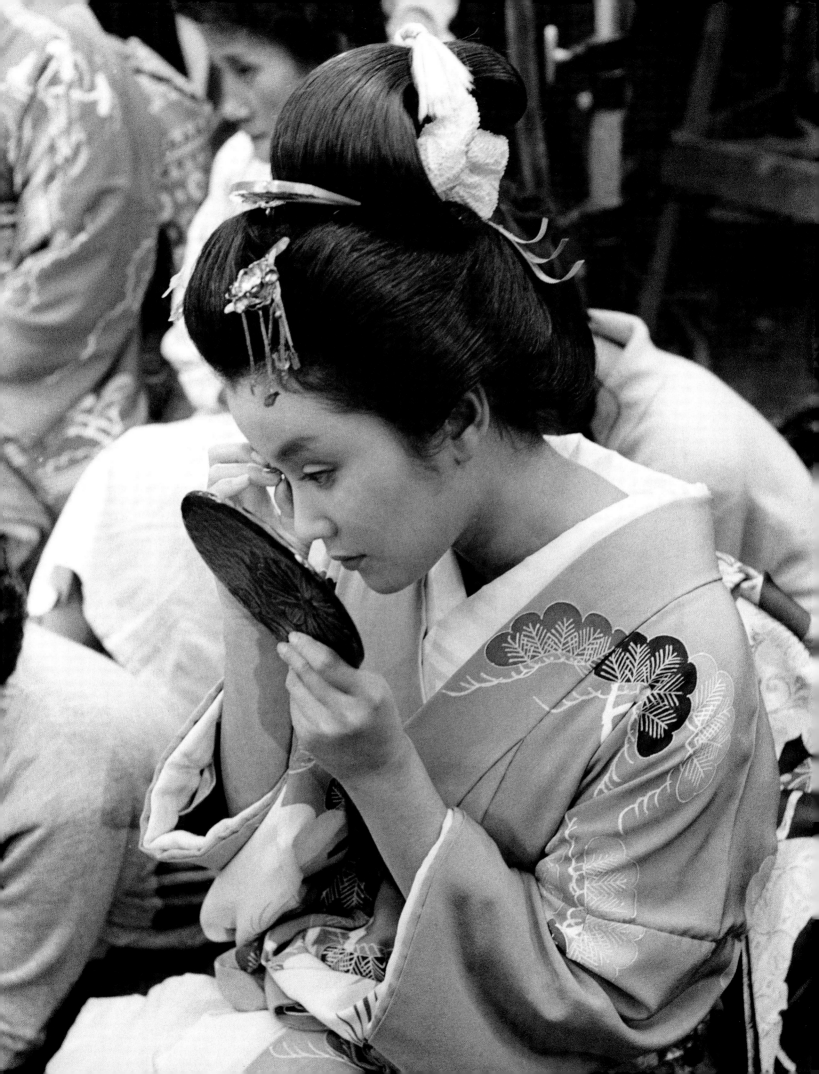

In 1935, Elizabeth Arden gave advice on beauty care for eyebrows and lashes. "Even if you do not make up your brows and lashes during the day, you should brush them carefully. A touch of Regenerator will make them shiny and silky and will do them a world of good. If your lashes are sparse and pale, the New Eyelash Cosmetic will make them darker and lovelier, and will also help you curl them." It came in Brown, Dark Brown, Black, Blue and Green. There was also a long-lasting "indelible cosmetic," which was perfectly waterproof, and suitable for smart or casual wear. This one was only available in Brown and Black.

Max Factor's "Color Harmony" system matched five natural eyelash and eyebrow colors to five eyebrow-pencil colors and three shades of mascara. Whatever your natural color, three colors were recommended for evening wear: green, blue and Riviera blue.

At the end of her career, Helena Rubenstein was still marveling at the truly fantastic products which lengthen the eyelashes infinitesimally with every application . . . rather like the droplets that extend the stalactite!

Traditionally, eye make-up has always been applied with sticks or pencils, which move toward the eye as if to penetrate its surface. A gesture with obvious erotic overtones . . . Nowadays, there appears to be a reversal of this inward movement, with the eyelashes sticking out horizontally like a row of spikes.

However, this outward movement does not necessarily imply aggressivity. In fact, made-up eyelashes now draw even more attention to the eye, surrounding it with an enticing fringe which is also far from innocent.

Twiggy: the flower eye of the flower-power era on the cover of *Vogue* (left). Right: The candor behind the mascara and false eyelashes, captured by Burt Glinn, December 1966.

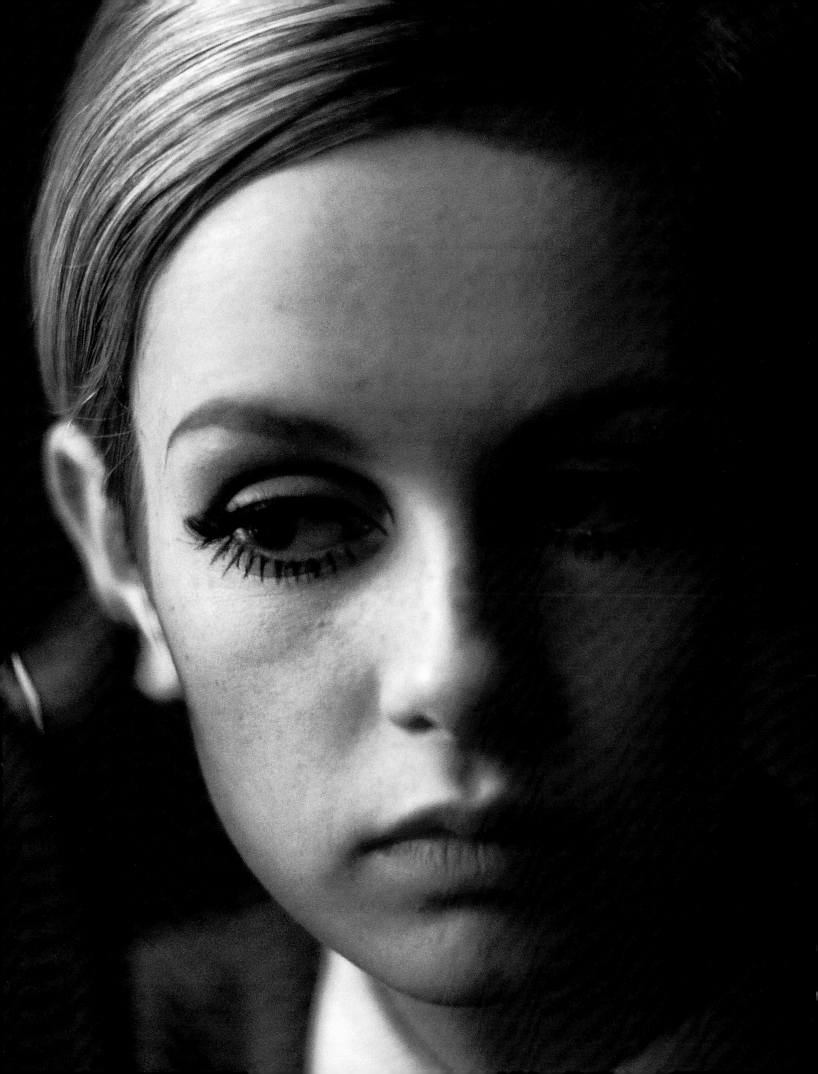

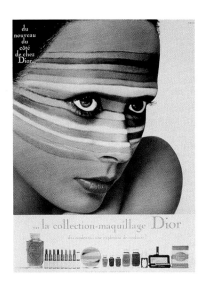

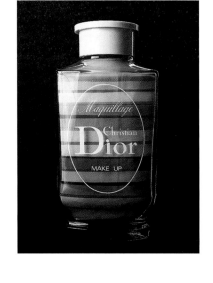

The beginnings of
Dior make-up, with the
"Explosion of Colors" in
1969: eyeshadow, nail
enamel, foundation and
lipstick . . . not to mention
blusher and mascara.
The stoppered bottle in which
the colors of this first range
are preserved (above).

Coming out
of the dark

Eye make-up gradually acquired a
wider range of colors—and one of
the positive results of this is that
women who paint their eyes are no
longer compared to chimney-sweeps
or coal merchants!

In the fourth century, Saint John
Chrysostom described eyebrows
that were so sooty "that they looked
as if they had been blackened with
the soot from a cooking pot," and
people were still being witty on the
subject in the 1920s, according to
the following account by Pringué:
"The countess Sommi-Piccinardi,
née Terra-Nova, arrived very late (at
the duchess of Camastra's
residence)—for she lived only at
night and had her tea when most
people dine—dressed in black as
always, with her face a glossy white,
her eyes ringed in thick black
make-up; this inspired the military

attaché to the British embassy to
say: 'We can supply coal to nobody,
as it is all reserved for the countess
Sommi-Piccinardi's eyes.'"

Things gradually became more
colorful, and by the time Elizabeth
Arden had created her eyeshadow
(Sha-do), all the colors of the
rainbow could be used to tint the
eyelids. "If your eyes are slightly
hazel or green, try a touch of green
Sha-do on your lids." In powder
form, it came in five colors: two
blues, two browns, and a chestnut.
The cream shadow range included
sixteen different shades: sky blue,
raven blue, black, gray, purple, light
brown, dark brown, dark chestnut,
green, moss green, light green, blue-
green, periwinkle, bronze, gold and
silver. In Max Factor's Color
Harmony table, there were only four
eyeshadow colors to match the four
identified eye colors.

In 1969, Dior launched his first

complete make-up line: the Explosion of Colors, including many shades of turquoise for the eyelids. Not long after, a new range followed, in a splash of bold colors like Mongol riders tearing across the steppes of central Asia: these were "the Tartars," six individual shades and four miniature palettes with four colors each. The violet-blue palette was called "the 205"—and despite its unimaginative name, it was a best-seller in duty-free shops for fifteen years, although elsewhere it was superseded by brown, gray and plum. Perhaps the 205 was particularly suited to the "flighty" eyes of long-distance travelers! In the fall of 1988, the palettes added a fifth color to their range, and one of them inherited the name "205." But—on the ground at any rate—eyeshadow colors were toning down, and getting darker again: they are shadows, after all.

Lip contour pencils,
By Terry.

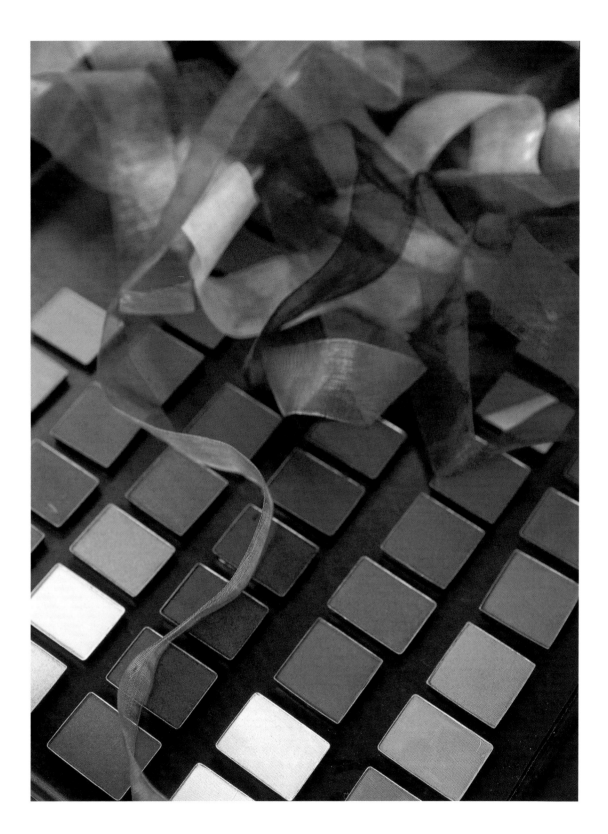

In the color laboratory
of Dior Perfumes: the
search for harmony and
coordination in fashion
and make-up—or the
perfect match of colors
and materials.
Right: the Fantastics,
a line of make-up created
for Dior by Serge Lutens,
fall-winter 1978.

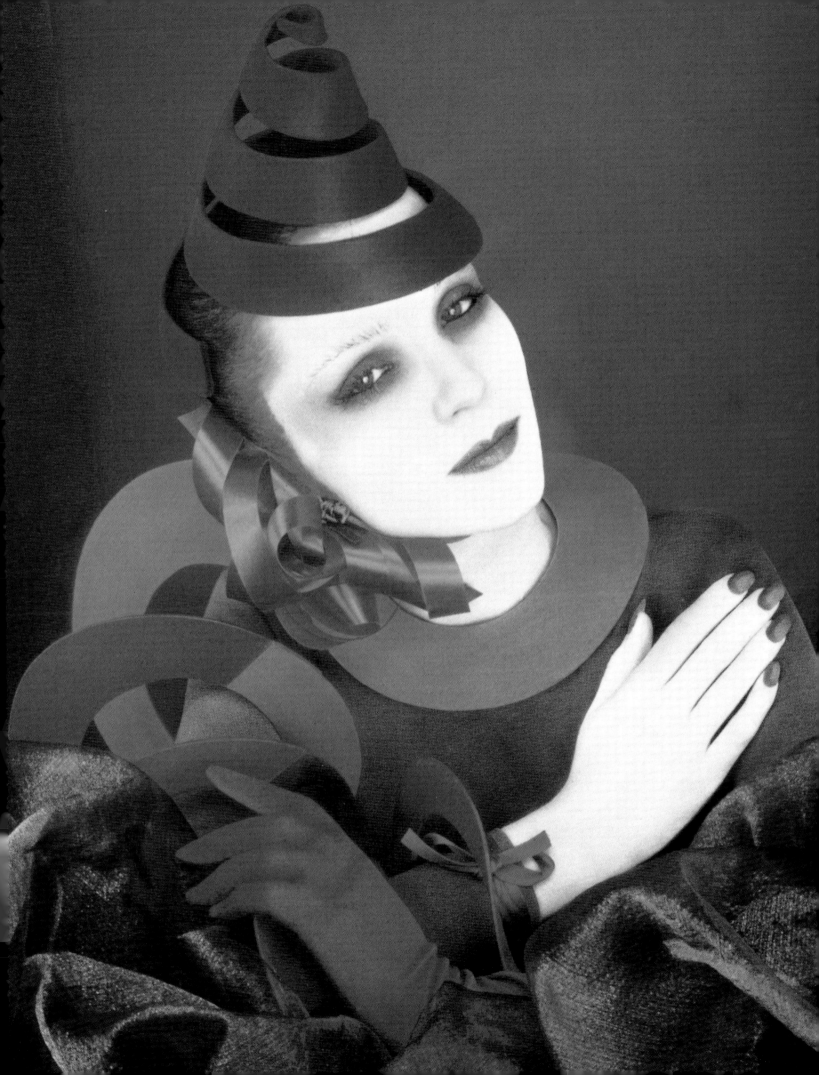

The mouth

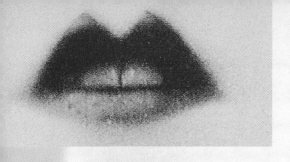

the keynote

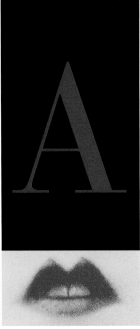

After white, used on the skin, and black to outline the eyes, red for lips and cheeks is the third fundamental color of make-up, and probably the color most commonly applied to the human body and inanimate objects. Seventy-thousand-year-old fragments of cosmetic rouge have been found on sites of Neanderthal settlements in East Africa. For thousands of years, red ocher was sprinkled on the skin of corpses or on their bones stripped of skin and flesh to prevent them from decomposing. It was also used on offerings.

In Asia, the color red has always represented creative or sexual power, life, light and happiness. The only trace of color that has come down to us from Neolithic Japan, between 3000 and 2000 B.C., is red ocher; funerary objects, such as the urns containing bodies or earthenware offerings, were painted with it. Today still, at the Sanno-sama shrine,

women spread a red-ocher powder on the open legs of statuettes of a female monkey representing a god.

In the Mediterranean world, the Egyptians, the Assyrians, the Greeks and the Romans all painted statues red. Among certain tribes in black Africa, rouge is applied over the bodies of the sick as a healing practice. Red, the color of blood, expresses the presence or permanence of life.

"She's a female. And all females are poison. They're full of wicked wiles."
Grumpy in
Snow White and the Seven Dwarfs

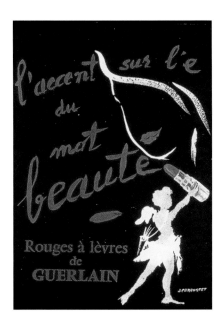

Guerlain advertisement, 1950s.
Right: Diorific Plastic Shine or "How to give life a shine" (Spring 1999). Photograph by Tyen. The mouth seems to stand out on the page, like a collage on the canvas of the skin or a pinned butterfly.
Preceding page: The sensual mouth of Jeanne Aubert in *Un joli monde*, a film directed by René Le Henaff, 1935.

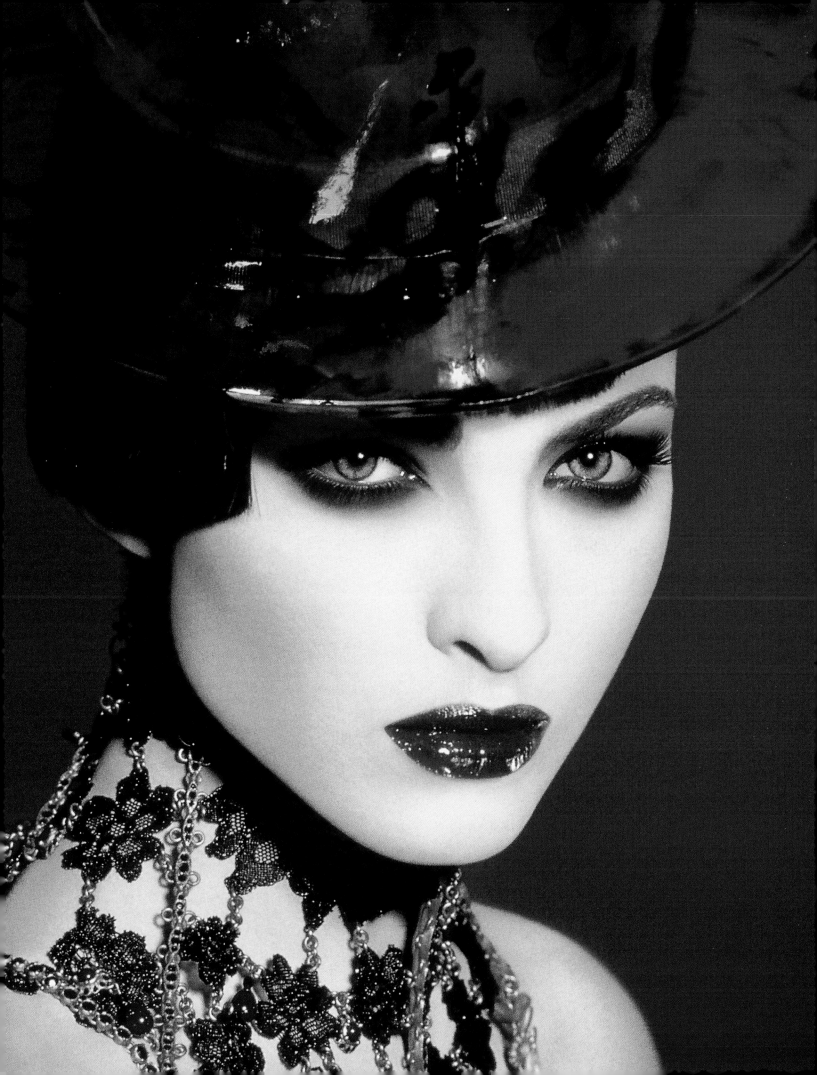

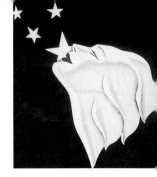

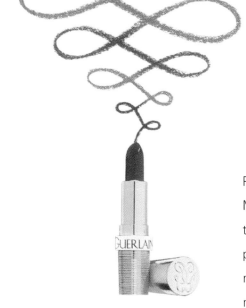

Kisskiss Douceur,
one of Guerlain's latest
lipsticks (above).
Top right: Advertisement
for a Guerlain lipstick.
Poster by J. Darcy, 1950s.

It is also a sign of sin: in the Passions of the twelfth century, Mary Magdalene buys rouge with the admitted aim of seducing young people, and a devil brings Mary a mirror to help her put on her make-up. In Renaissance theater, Concupiscence and Infidelity often advise Mary to whiten her dark complexion, dye her hair yellow and paint her lips red. Associated with sin, make-up was even the instrument of the ensuing punishment; there are numerous stories of poisoned cosmetics in the tragedies of Jacobean England. Lucrezia Borgia makes herself up on stage with cosmetics sent by her lover, which disfigure her, and there are similar episodes in Christopher Marlowe's *Dr Faustus*, in six of Ben Johnson's plays and in John Webster's *The White Devil*.

While white often represents the virginal or the angelic,

red evokes violent images: St. John Chrysostom mocked "blood-red lips like the scarlet jaws of a bear," and Juvenal wondered, "is it a face or a wound?"

Philostratus the Lemnian handled bloody images with the delicacy of a gardener and compared lips to "the blood of roses." A description by Gabriel-Louis Pringué runs as follows: "Venice was filled with the fragrance of tuberose and gardenia, mingled with the melancholic, damp, insipid smell of the canals . . . A dead woman entered. Her superb figure was molded in a white satin dress draped like a shroud with a long train; a clump of orchids hid her breast. Her hair was red; her alabaster-white, green-veined face was consumed by two enormous eyes, whose black contours almost reached the mouth, which was painted a red so dark that it resembled a cake of coagulated

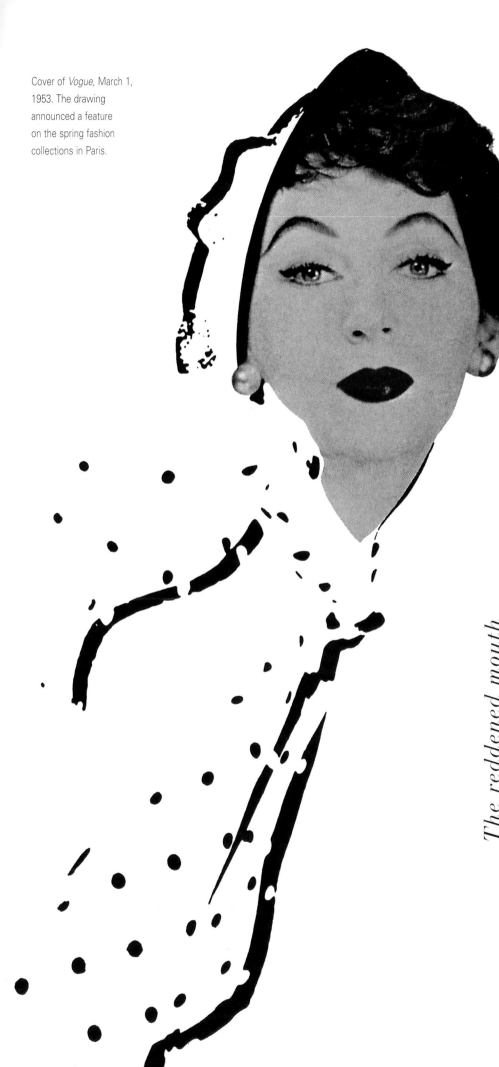

Cover of *Vogue*, March 1, 1953. The drawing announced a feature on the spring fashion collections in Paris.

The reddened mouth

Vermilion is generally made from powdered cinnabar, a natural mercuric sulfide mined around the Mediterranean from the foot of the Caucasus to the Iberian peninsula. Red lead oxide (or minium) is artificial and obtained from ceruse, a natural lead carbonate. Murex purple comes from the thick spiny shell of shellfish found on the islands off the ancient Mauretania of King Juba and in present-day Essaouira.

Carmine is obtained from the female cochineal insect. "Vegetable" cinnabar is extracted from the dragon tree of the Canary Islands and Brazil; its bark exudes a sort of resin, dragon's blood, which becomes crumbly and blood red on drying. The root of the anchusa or alkanet of the borage family, found in all southern and arid regions of Europe and in the rocky ground of southern France, yields a dark-red coloring matter. Fucus is obtained from marine seaweed such as kelp and wrack. Wine lees are also used. Finally, throughout the Muslim world the habit of chewing betel to color the gums and lips an attractive red has existed for centuries; no other make-up is used.

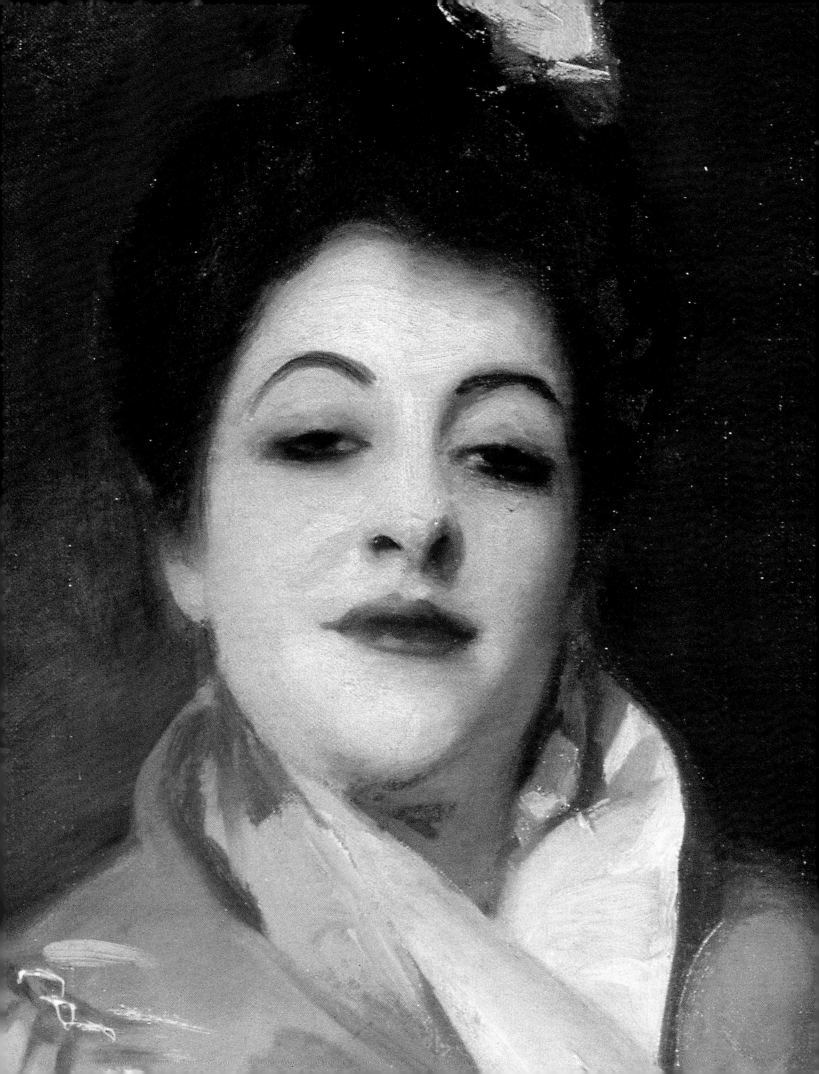

blood. She carried a very young leopard in her arms. It was the Marquise Casati." She would be painted by Kees Van Dongen.

White turned woman into a statue; red made the marble bleed, opening the mouth-wound, revealing the aperture, placing sexuality right in the middle of the face under the eyes of the soul.

Yukio Mishima describes the moment when he came face to face with his distant relative Chako, a woman five years' his elder: "When I saw her too-red lips, I felt embarrassed and fell silent. Perhaps it was because of my fever, but that crimson color seemed to bore into my eyes and gave me a violent headache. 'You put on so much,' I said to her. 'How can you put on so much make-up at such a time without people in the street commenting? . . . ' At that moment, my feverish breathing mingled with hers. My lips were covered with something thick and greasy."

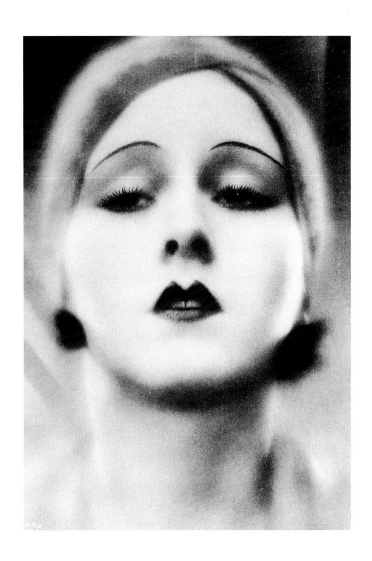

The mouth

The "woman machine" of the 1920s photographed by Anon for an advertisement for G. Mandel (above). By Terry's Rouge Terriblement Rouge ("the color of the great seductresses") lipstick and Rouge Précis nail enamel (right). Left: All pallor, blood red and gold, *La Carmencita* (detail) by John Singer Sargent, 1892.

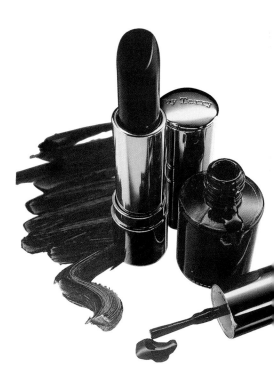

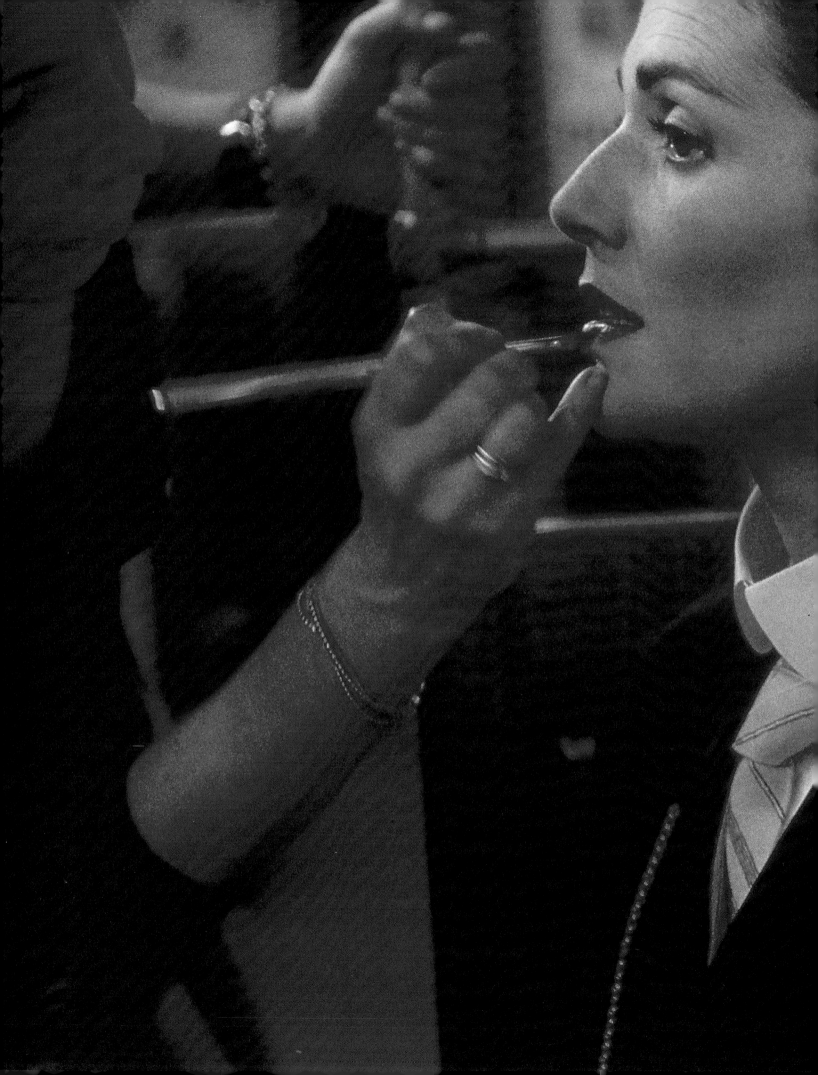

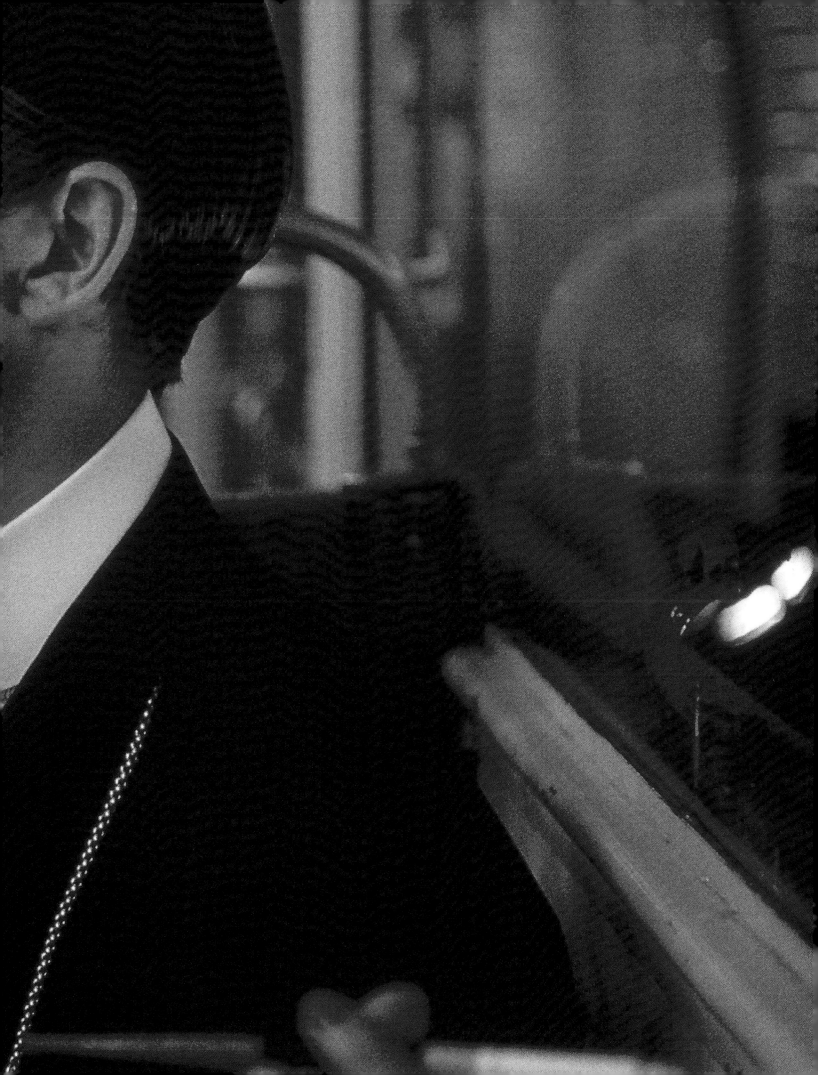

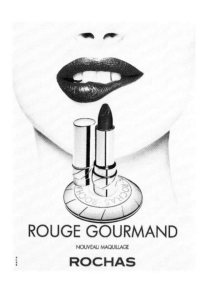

ROUGE GOURMAND

NOUVEAU MAQUILLAGE

ROCHAS

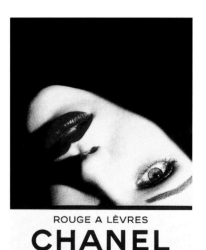

ROUGE A LÈVRES

CHANEL

Lipstick kiss

Lipstick—which is not necessarily so "greasy"—is, of course, closely connected to kissing. Royal connoisseur Lola Montès, favorite of King Ludwig of Bavaria (perhaps the monarch was, in this respect, the equal of Louis XV?) maintained that lipstick was incompatible with kissing: "There is no man who would not shrink back in disgust at the idea of a kiss from a pair of painted lips!"

But this is not necessarily so. The prostitute who meets Mishima knew how to counteract disgust: "Clasping her to me, I made to kiss her. Then her heavy shoulders began to shake wildly with laughter. 'Don't do that. You'll put lipstick everywhere. This is how to do it.' The prostitute opened her large mouth with gold teeth, framed with lipstick, and stuck out a thick rod-like tongue. Following her example, I stuck out mine. The ends of our tongues met . . ."

A symbolic inversion of the sexes might be seen in this image, echoed in today's trend in make-up of accentuating the fullness of the lips, highlighting the relief of the mouth and emphasizing its curves and convexity.

The fact remains that, far from discouraging kisses, lipstick attracts them, whether the lips are fleshy or not. "And the lips!" exclaims Morin. "Those of Joan Crawford are stenciled over millions of others throughout the world. The natural mouth withdraws behind a second mouth, bloody and triumphant, ceaselessly repainted to elicit the mental kiss of the passer-by."

Beyond its role as a fantasy-teaser, lipstick is sold in a very down-to-earth manner as "the way to get your claws into him," the lasso with which to catch a husband. When Max Factor, whose principal advertising emblem was Joan Crawford, launched the new color Ruban Corail in his Colorfast line of creamy, glossy and long-

Two advertising visuals of the 1990s: Chanel's temptress mouth (above) and Rochas' greedy lips, 1992 (top). Preceding pages: a model being made up during the season's ready-to-wear collection fashion show, Paris, 1994.

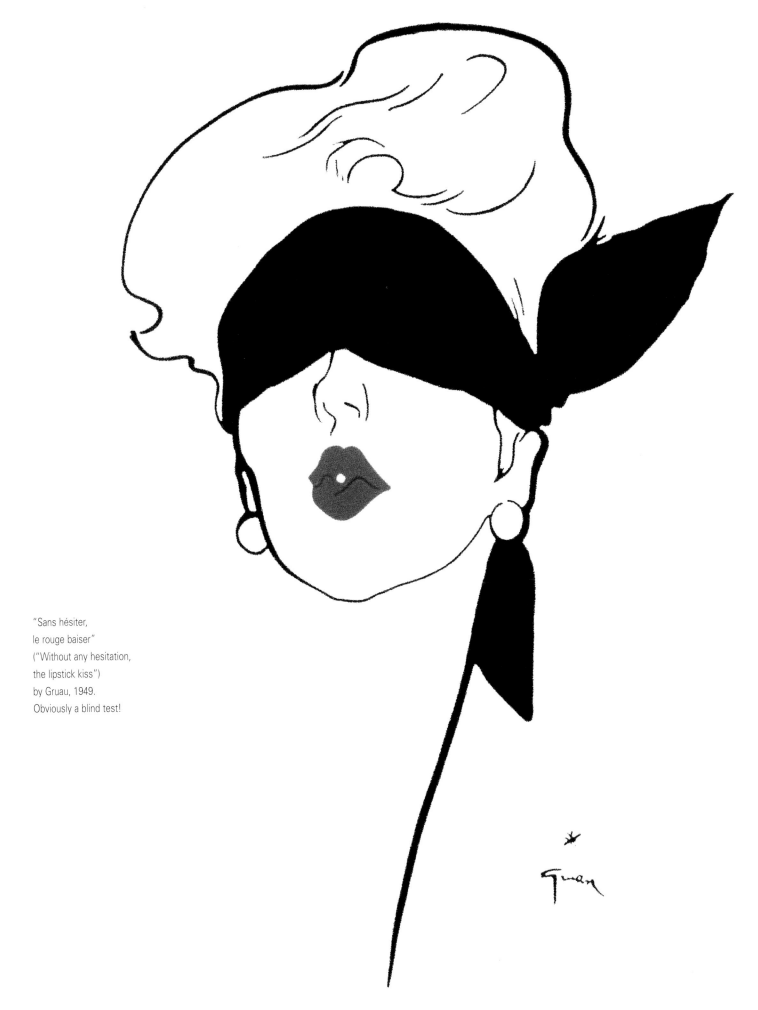

"Sans hésiter,
le rouge baiser"
("Without any hesitation,
the lipstick kiss")
by Gruau, 1949.
Obviously a blind test!

Below right: Teenage love in
Mystery Train a film by
Jim Jarmusch, 1989. "She
who over-kisses kills a
man's desire . . ."
Below: Limited edition of a
solid-silver powder compact
and lipstick case created by
the silversmith Georg Jensen
for Shu Uemura.
Right: The moving beauty of
Florette in a play of shadow
and light, photographed
by Jacques-Henri Lartigue,
January 1944.

lasting lipsticks, he described it as
"A 'fashion' shade that matches
the colors used in haute-couture,
and most of all, a color that gives
your lips that fascinating sheen
which catches men's eyes and
invites a kiss." The clearly stated
slogan of the publicity campaign
was "Keep him for ever"; the
visual showed a man held on a
"coral-ribbon" leash by a woman.

Forty years later, Revlon was
still selling the ColorStay brand as
"a long-lasting kiss-resistant lipstick
that doesn't leave marks." "At love
school, all kisses are permitted
with ColorStay lipliner by Revlon:
it can keep a secret in all
circumstances! . . . It neither stains
nor leaves marks on glasses,
teeth, or . . . the man of your life!

With ColorStay lipliner, you'll see
how simple it is to make a success
of your make-up and transform your
mouth into a kissing-magnet!"
And at the end of the kiss, there's
the husband, as a description of
rival products makes clear:
"Unfortunately, their benefits often
disappear as quickly as the luster
of their color . . . and the expected
'glamour' effect vanishes along with
the wearer's highest hopes . . ."
(an expression that always
signified matrimonial expectations).
The advertising line for mass-
produced lipstick is still centered
on the concept of lipstick-as-bait
that ends with a ring on the finger;
Bourjois' pink from the Éclat de
Rire collection "makes us happy
and attracts kisses . . ."

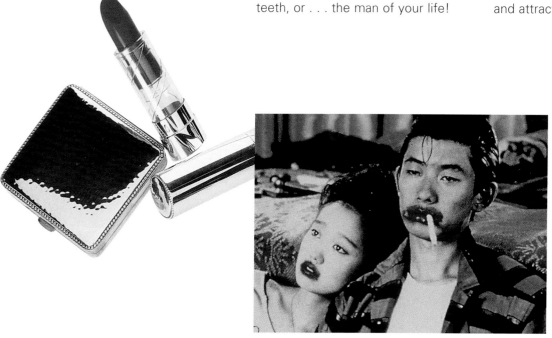

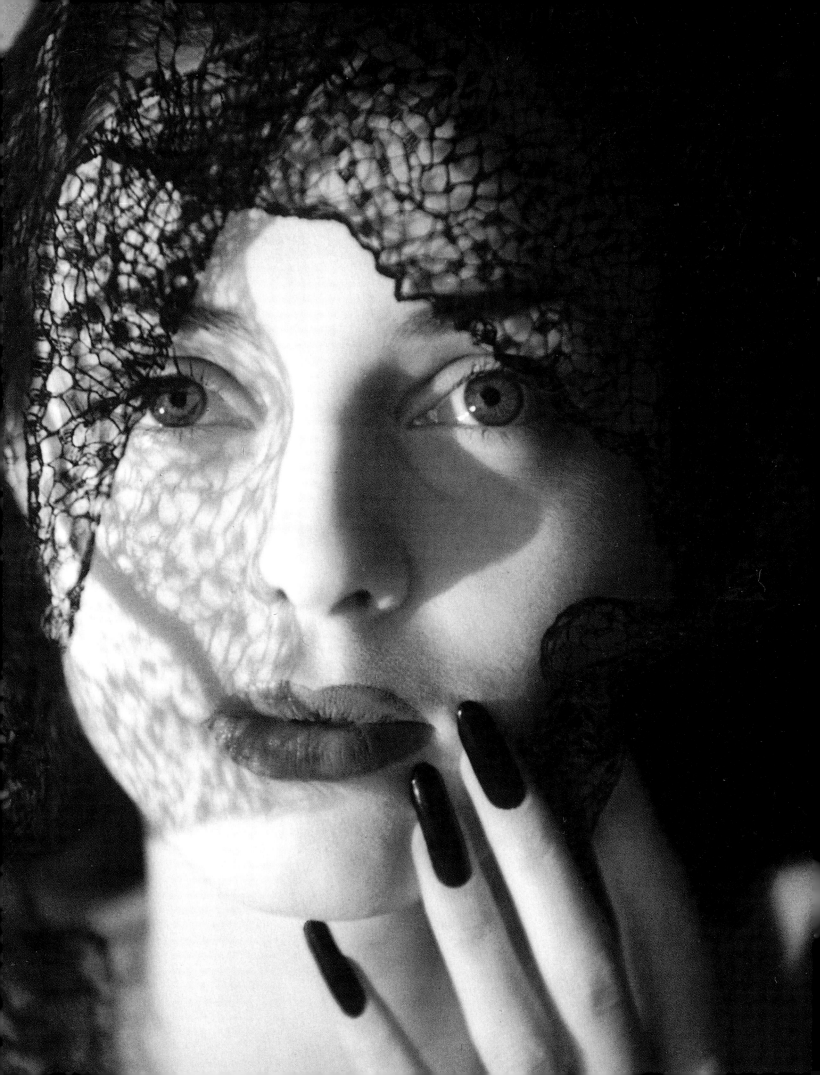

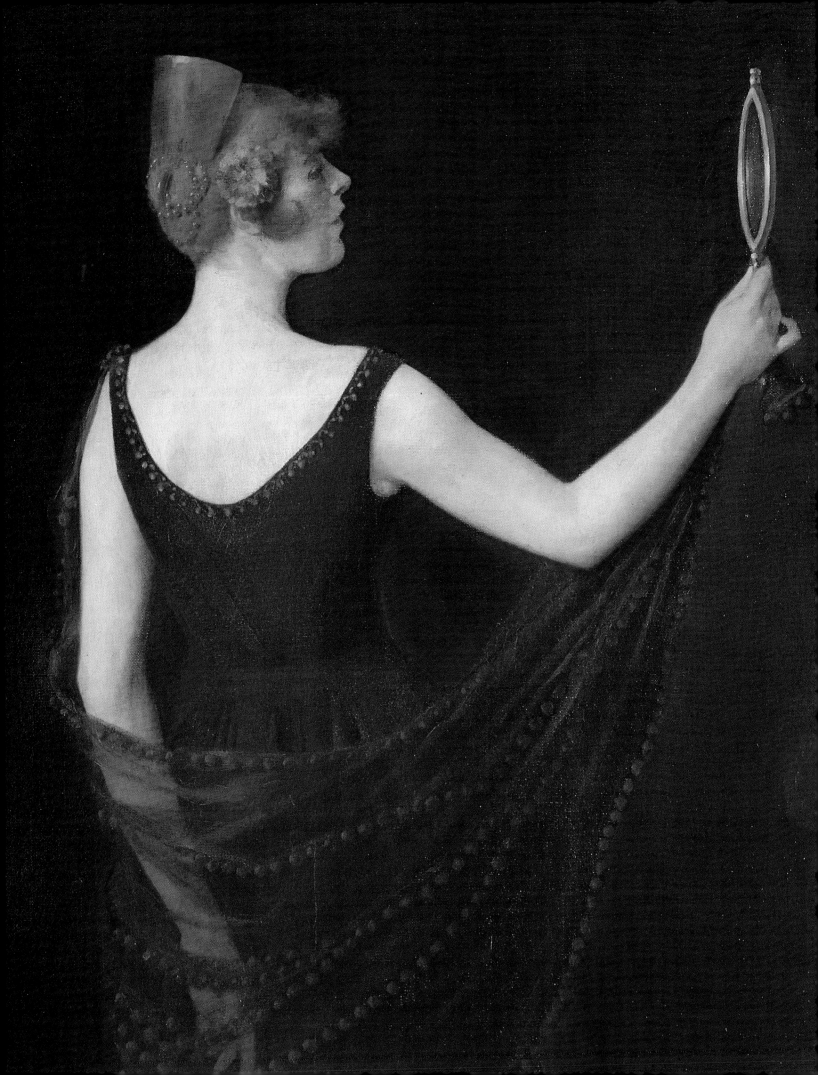

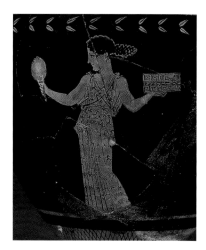 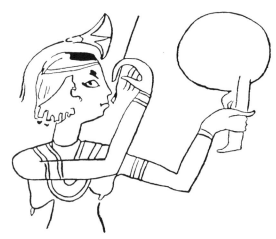

Self-love and mirror play

Luxury lipstick advertising tends to center on autoeroticism: the love story is between oneself and one's make-up; the kiss is given to one by one's lipstick. One of Guerlain's lipsticks is called Kisskiss—the name is a pleonasm, a kiss repeated; yet there is never a question of kissing in the advertising: "Kisskiss Douceur has an incomparable slippery silky effect. It is applied voluptuously . . . A delicious sensation . . . Sensual skin with new suppleness . . . A comforting sensation that promises permanent well-being. Its fine, soft texture is a delight!" You dress yourself with it as if it were a second skin, slip voluptuously into it, feel its caress on your skin: it's the lipstick kissing you!

It is also a product for women who enjoy their food: lipstick is a lollipop, an ice cream, something to taste. In 1998, the Lipshine lip glosses were presented as candy with names such as Barley Sugar, Toffee, Candy, and Marshmallow.

When the Church condemned the use of make-up, it declared that women should carefully shut themselves away during this operation so that no one should disturb them. If they have to hide, is it not because they know that they are guilty? Guilty only of resorting to artifice, or guilty of indulging in autoeroticism with only their mirror or female companions as witnesses?

Narcissism has always required a mirror. The Chinese woman held a polished bronze mirror in her left hand by the knob in the center,

The satirical papyrus of the Egyptian Museum in Turin (above), and *Woman with a Mirror* holding a make-up box, a red-figure skyphos, 420–410 B.C. (above left). Left: A mirror, a kiss curl, a dress like a theater curtain . . . Vision, seduction, representation: the picture says it all. *The Woman in Red* by William T. Dannat, 1889.

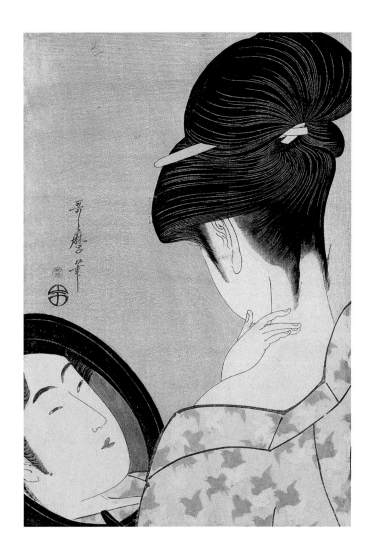

Woman Applying Make-up,
Kitagawa Utamaro,
late eighteenth century.
Engraver of the lives of the
women of Edo, Utamaro
spent most of his time in
Yoshiwara, the "the nightless
city." He invented the
close-up of face and upper
bust within the *ukiyo-e* genre,
and created the illusion of
multiple reflections.
Right: *Renée* by
Jacques-Henri Lartigue,
Basque region, 1930.

like a lid, from which hung a tassel, turning it over to apply red paste to her lips.

The Greek woman's mirror was enclosed in a round, *repoussé* bronze box. Aphrodite was sometimes depicted on the handle, standing naked on a squatting lion and flanked by two mermaids. The mirror reflected the woman's use of the wonderful red make-up of Sinope, city of Asia Minor on the Black Sea whose name came from that of an Amazon queen. The lady of Tanagra's polished-metal mirror was held in the center of her feather fan. The lady would have used vermilion extracted from the silver mines of Colchis or Spain.

The Egyptian woman used a mirror of bronze with incrustations of electrum, a natural alloy of gold and silver found in the sands of the Pactolus River in ancient Lydia. She would probably not usually have made up her mouth, yet a caricature on the satirical papyrus from the New Kingdom period in the Turin museum shows a woman (of easy virtue?) painting her lips. In any case, pressed by her over-impatient lover, this lady only mentions eye make-up: "He does not let me get a dress, / nor carry my fan; / He no longer lets me put make-up on my eyes, / or use any perfume!"

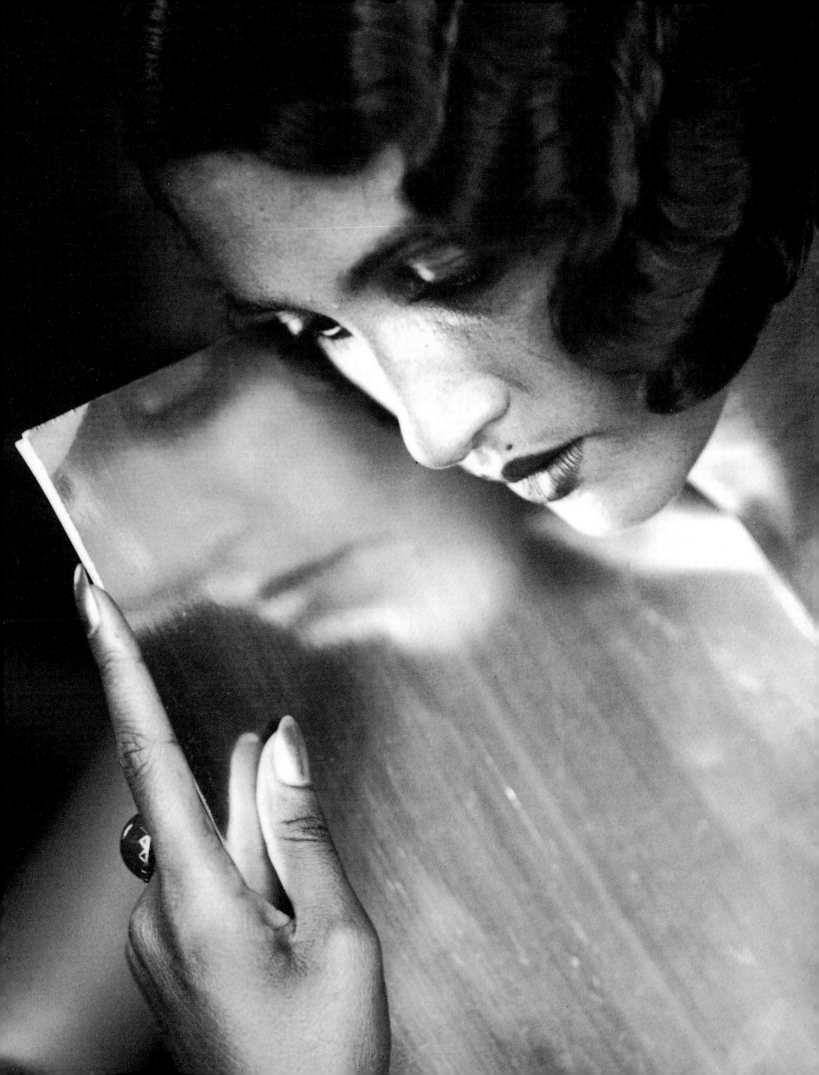

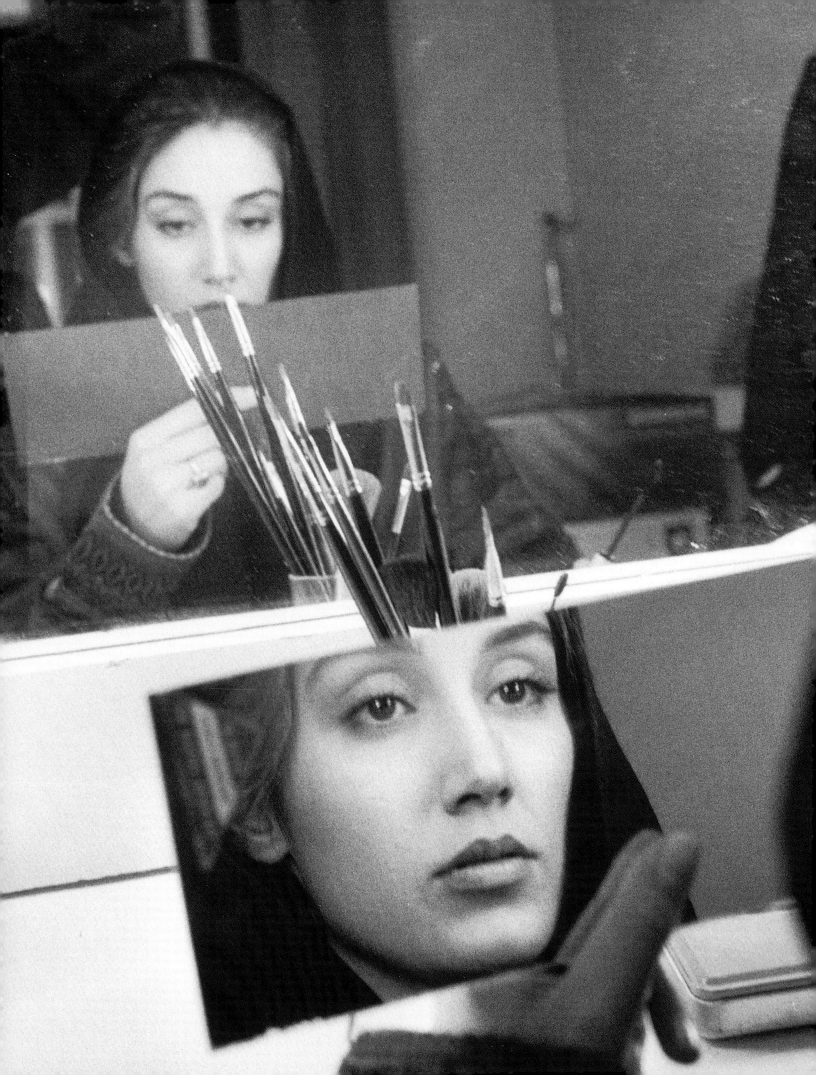

A mirror with a carved ivory handle buried in lava by Mount Vesuvius in A.D. 79 bears witness to the direct relations between India, from where the mirror came, and Pompeii. With the aid of a little spatula, the *miltos*, its lovely owner would have applied a red ocher to her lips, clay reddened by natural iron oxide or obtained artificially from burnt yellow ocher.

In Mexico, the Aztec woman's mirror was made of obsidian or volcanic glass, black, vitreous magma rock; or of crystalline marcasite, a natural iron sulfide, with an engraving on the back representing Eecatl, god of wind; or of pyrite, a copper sulfide that looks very much like gold. "Listen, my daughter, you must never paint your mouth to be beautiful" might have said a member of the ruling classes in Tenochtitlan, Mexico.

In the Middles Ages, the mirrors were made of gold and silver, or steel, imported from Damascus, which supplied men with blades and women with their reflection. At the same time, a tinctorial wood, red as glowing embers, whence its name, *braisil*, was imported from India. In 1556 it gave its name to that region of South America whose forests are full of it.

From the fifteenth century on, mirrors were made of a thin sheet of glass covered with a strip of metal— silvered mirrors— a process that spread from Germany to Venice. It was before Venetian mirrors that the French woman made herself up until the seventeenth century. Then the royal factory at last began to produce perfectly colorless and polished mirror glass, which definitively replaced metal.

Metal and beauty are as inseparable from each other as a mirror and its silvering: in the central room of Castle Solitude in Stuttgart, where twelve groups of divinities depict the industries and riches of Württemberg, Venus and the Graces symbolize the country's mirror factories. When the duke installed his mistress, Wilhelmine von Grävenitz, at the Jägerhaus in Stuttgart in 1707, he offered her a mirror-lined boudoir.

"And lips become a mirror . . . with Diorific Plastic Shine. Incredibly smooth, polished, ultra-shiny. However they move, reflections play continuously over their convex form." This is the definitive moment of narcissism. Before her mirror, the woman is herself a reflector in a play of mirrors, in which her image is reflected to infinity.

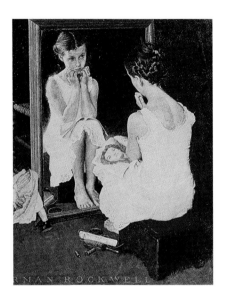

Difficult to be a star . . . Dreaming before her own reflection, Norman Rockwell's *The Girl at the Mirror* searches for her identity (cover of the *Morning Post*, March 1954). Left: The young Iranian actress Hedieh Tehrani, unveiled, during the filming of *Shokaran*, a film directed by Behrouz Afkhami, 1998.

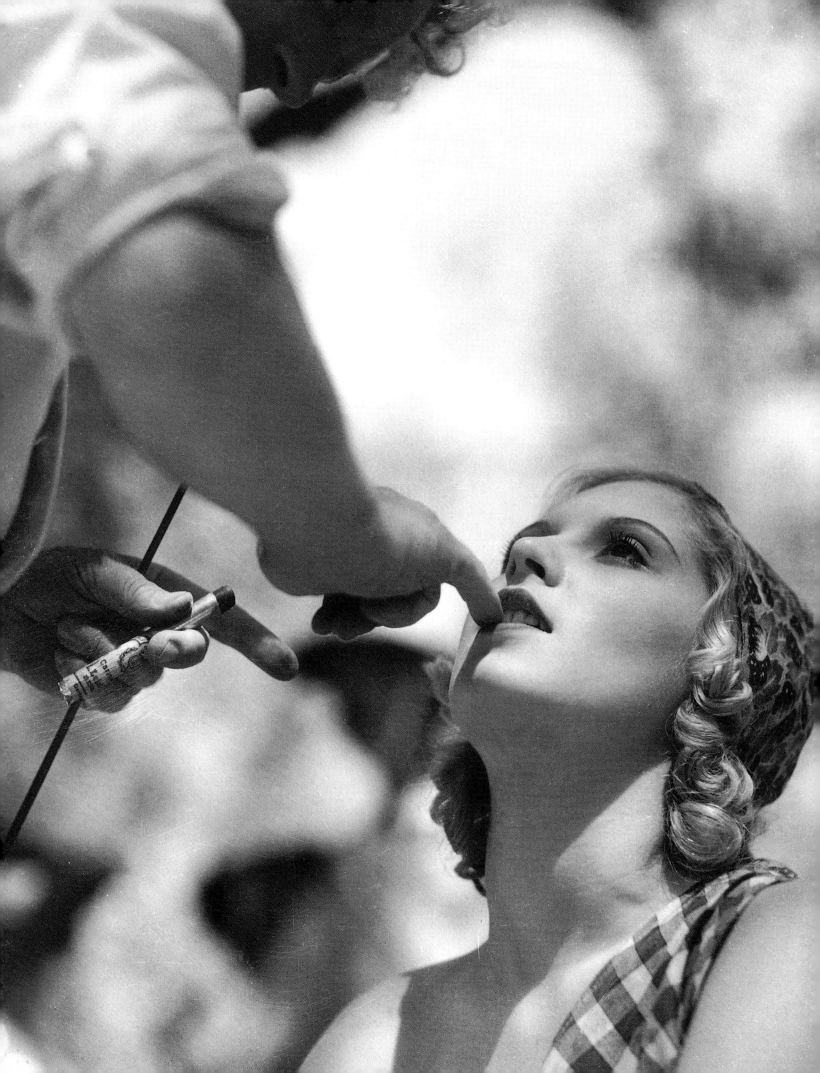

By word of mouth

The mouth speaks, to say the least. It most often communicates the ritual or social, but not always through red. According to Lane, women of the highest classes in Upper Egypt colored their lips in the manner of face and hand tattoos, which gave them a dark-blue tint, "extremely unpleasant to the foreign eye." "In Baghdad it is highly fashionable to paint the mouth blue," assures Mrs. Cocheris, "and in Aleppo, to blacken the gums and lips. The young girls of Sakatou dye their teeth, hands, nails and feet red. The girls of Nyfia do better still: through the use of caustics they manage to have blue hair and eyebrows, black eyelashes, yellow teeth, scarlet lips, hands and feet. It's the last word in elegance; rosy skin only excites pity, terror and astonishment. . . ."

Around 1810, it became fashionable among the geishas of Edo and the *onnagata*—men who performed the roles of courtesans in kabuki drama, and who were the

"Face. What did Permelle not try in order to give herself a small mouth and whiten her skin! She spent a third of her life in front of a mirror . . ." (Caraccioli, who described the customs of the century in his Dictionary)

"How far we have come since the little heart-shaped mouth of ladies in 1900! . . . After the refined curve of the lips of Clara Bow in the 1920s, it was Joan Crawford's admirable large mouth and the natural, expressive mouth of Audrey Hepburn. Women's mouths today are spontaneous, joyous, sensual and free" (Helena Rubinstein).

"When I returned to Paris in September 1929 I was carried away by my freedom. Every morning I put on my make-up with glamour and piquant: a thick red stroke on each cheekbone, lots of powder, red lipstick on my lips" (Simone de Beauvoir).

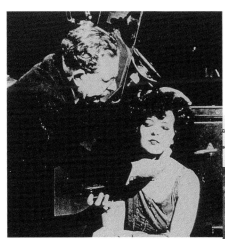

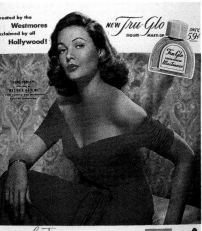

Left: Josette Day being made up during the shooting of *The Adventures of King Pausole* (1932). Photograph by Jacques-Henri Lartigue. The actress married a millionaire, Maurice Solvay, in 1950, and abandoned acting.

Max Factor, the make-up artist of the stars, and his model Clara Bow, 1920s (above). Thirty years later, Gene Tierney advertises a line of products created by the Westmore brothers, make-up artists in Hollywood ("guardian angels of the beauty of the stars") (right).

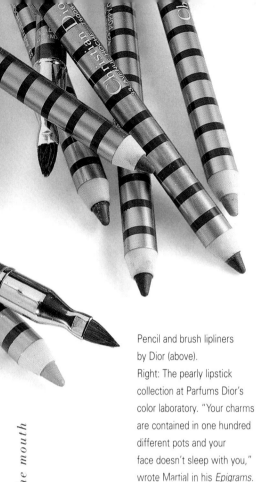

Pencil and brush lipliners by Dior (above).
Right: The pearly lipstick collection at Parfums Dior's color laboratory. "Your charms are contained in one hundred different pots and your face doesn't sleep with you," wrote Martial in his *Epigrams*.

arbiters of elegance in town—to apply green make-up to the lower lip.

In Italy, Thailand and South America today, the preference is for orange tints. Paler colors verging on beige are preferred in the United States; there is a tendency toward blue in Europe (except in Italy), and pink in the Nordic countries. Asia likes pearly lipsticks, but the Japanese hate pale pearly finishes.

The mouth is not just the lips. When the male Carib Indians go to war or wish to present a display of splendor, their women use genipap juice to give them mustaches. In the Kuril Islands near Japan, the young Ainu women draw a sort of red mustache above their upper lip. In the time of Louis XIV in France faces were studded with beauty spots. A spot on the corner of the mouth was called the *baiseuse* (kisser); when it was on the lips it was *friponne* (cheeky) or *coquette* (flirtatious), and when under the lower lip, it was *discrète* (discreet). Chinese women also put beauty spots on the side of their mouths.

The custom of dying teeth black or dark red with cochineal was widespread in Mesoamerica among the Huastecs (a tribe from the far north) and the Otomis (just north of the capital), and certain Mexican women adopted it in the sixteenth century, as recounted by the Franciscan Fray Bernardino de Sahagún.

In Japan in the nineteenth century, a custom among the nobility was for married women to blacken their teeth. Apprentice courtesans, the *kamuro*, entered the service of their mistress between five and seven years old. At the age of thirteen or fourteen, they became *shinzo* and blackened their teeth for the first time with hot iron trimmings that were thrown into water and mixed with oak-gall powder. This dental powder was called *haguro*. Goncourt reported that "a Japanese man can require a *Oiran* to blacken her teeth. The relationship then becomes a form of marriage that is valid in Yoshiwara, and the courtesan cannot accept a proposal from a serious friend, unless unknown to the man who paid for her to have her teeth blackened. Yes, she is not supposed to have any other relations."

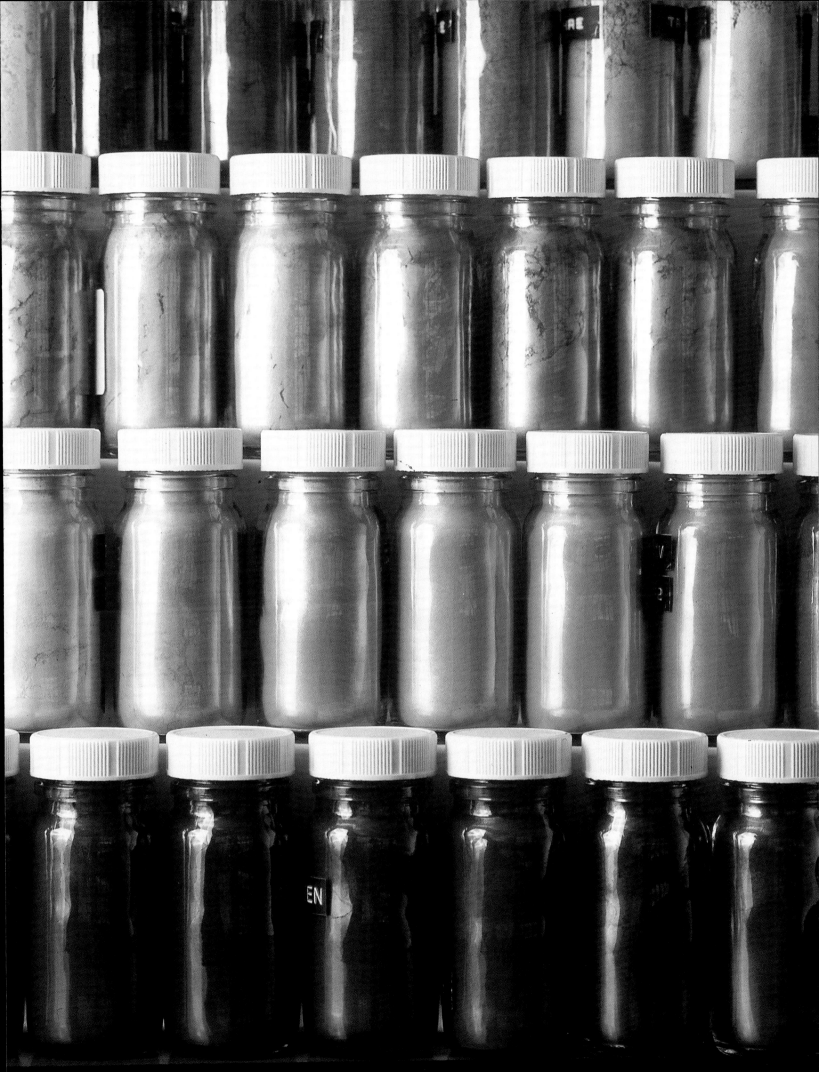

Lipsticks in all colors

For many years the mouth communicated the ritual, the fashionable and the social. Today it speaks of the individual. Éliane Gouriou, its "interpreter" at Dior, explains: "A fleshy mouth made up with matte beige means 'I do not want to be noticed for this aspect of my personality.' If it is made up with glossy cherry red, it means 'I have sensual and luscious lips, which I accept and which I offer.' If it is painted dark brown or violet, it says 'I provoke, I impose myself, but my mouth is not to be touched; what's more, men hate it'!"

Speaking all languages, communicating every frame of mind and the least change of mood, lip make-up could not restrict itself to red. Happy nineteenth century! Life naturally provided you with ruby lips; cosmetics were only used to repair a temporary fading of color. "Cherry-red ruby lips generally indicate perfect health. However, a healthy woman does not necessarily have beautiful lips. In this case, benzoin dye can be used," Lola Montès liked to say.

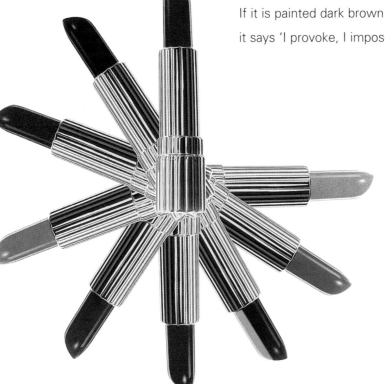

Rouge Diorific by
Christian Dior (below)
and Estée Lauder's Futurist
lipsticks (left).
Right: the lips' soldiers before
attack, by Shu Uemura.

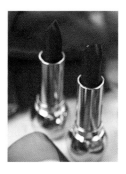

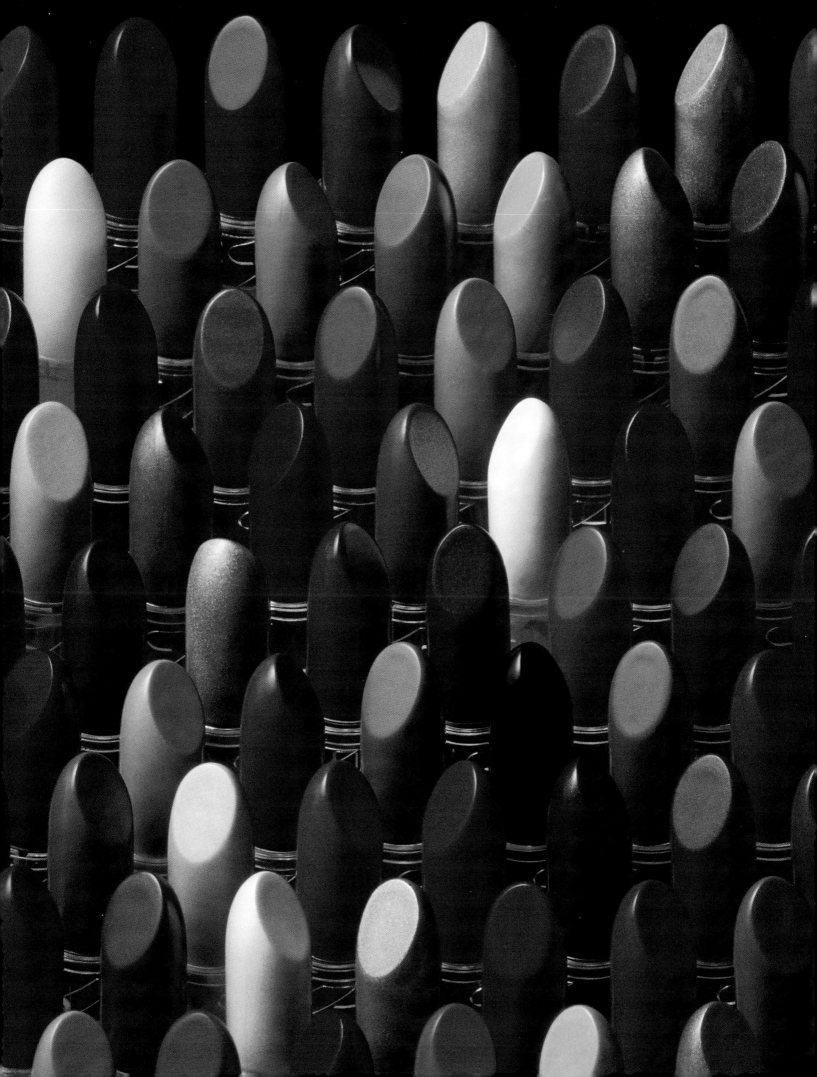

Lipstick manufacture at the Parfums Dior factory obeys strict and unchanging rules (below): the pigments are crushed and mixed with a waxy base, then homogenized in a vat at 85°C.

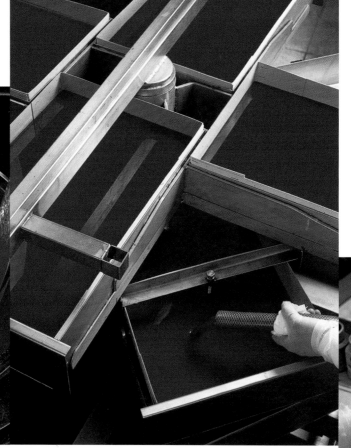

Color control tests and emptying of the vat containing the molten lipstick into individual containers to make bars (above), followed by pouring, which can be a manual or automatic operation. Right: checking the "bullets"—the lip "sticks"— on a production line.

Manual pouring: the lipstick
is poured into molds
(below left). The excess
paste (far right) is scraped
off with a spatula. The
"bullets" (below) are then
made and checked one by
one; those with defects
—an air bubble, for
example—are immediately
eliminated.

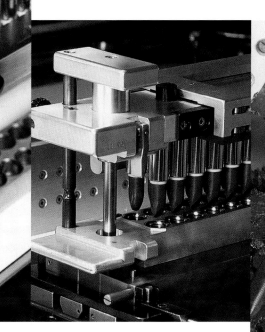

And the unique driving force
behind all this is "the desire
to please, the desire to
renew one's appearance,
in order to maintain or
renew the feelings of love"
Christian Dior.

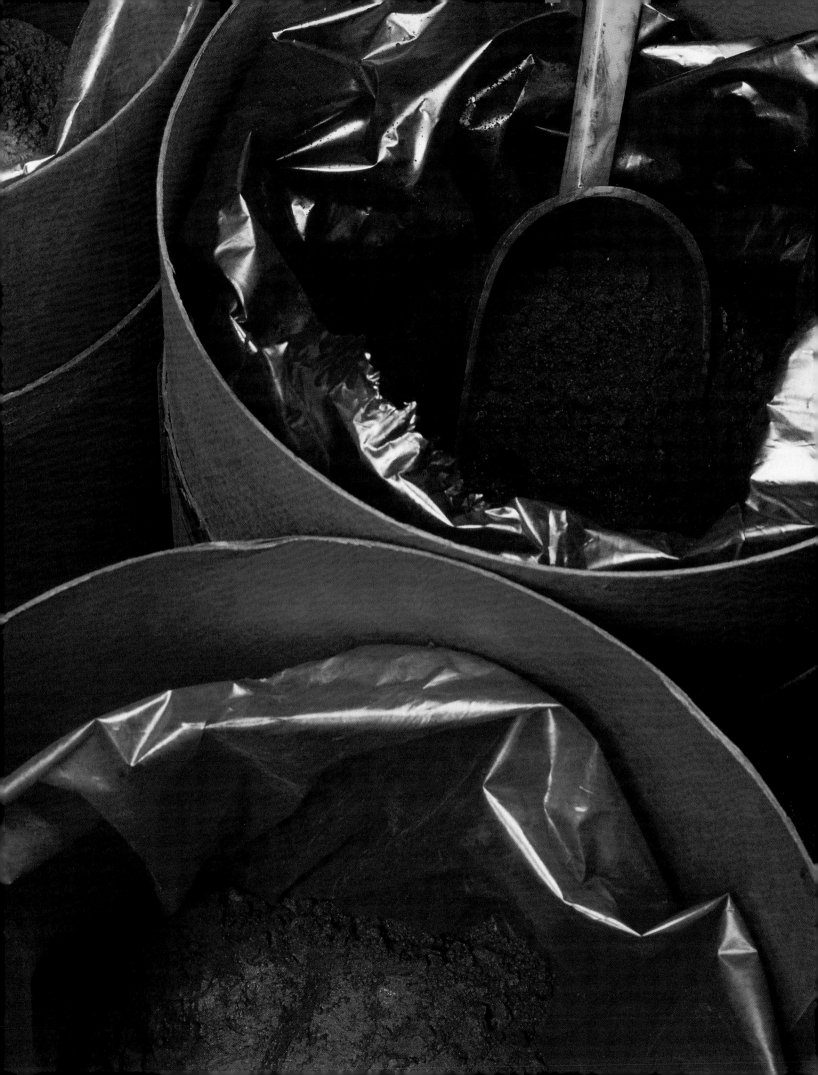

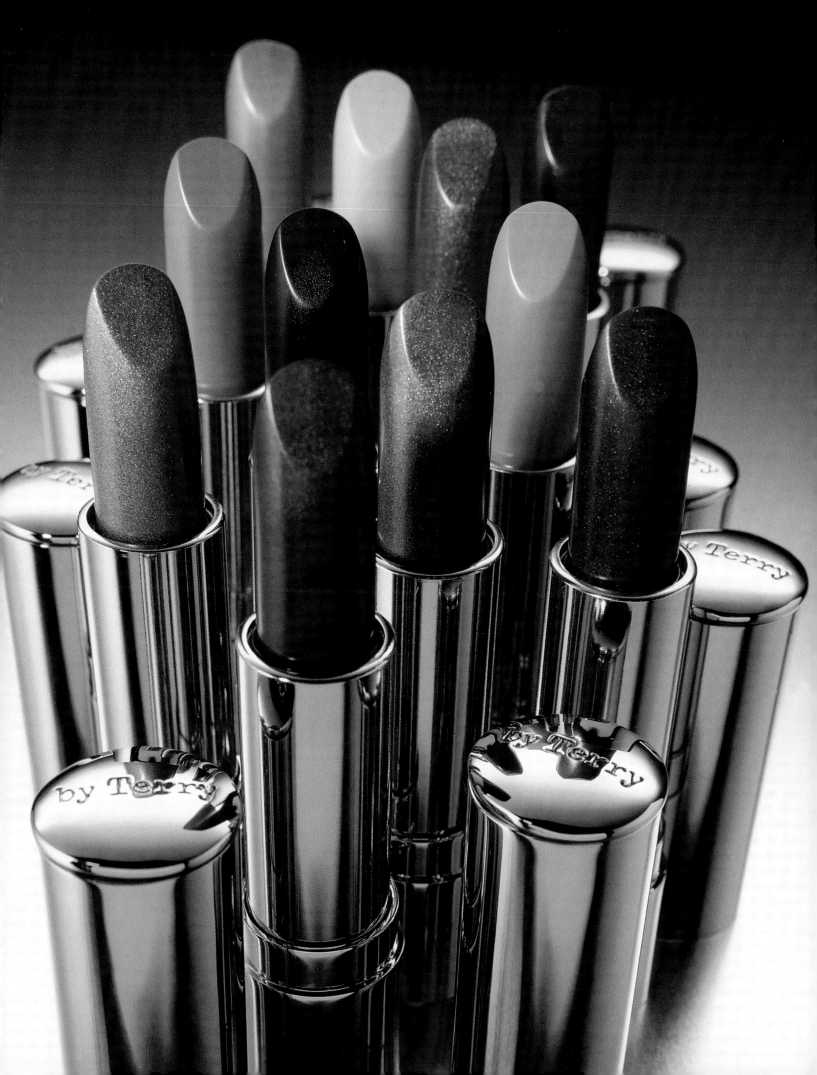

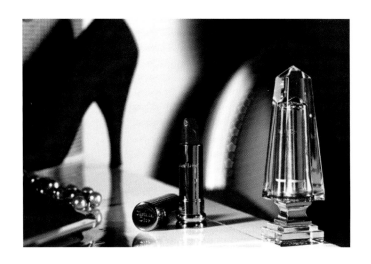

The three pillars of seduction:
lipstick, high heels and lipstick
again, in the form of a cut
crystal "obelisk case" for the
dressing table, Dior, 1955 (left).
The 1956 lipstick frame (below).

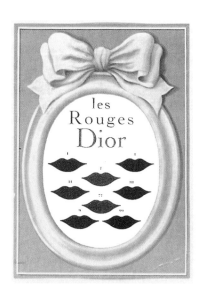

At the beginning of the 1920s lipstick began to be mass-distributed, perhaps because of a desire to display the gender differences that World War I had suppressed in fashion, uniform and the workplace: the elastic girdle had done away with the hourglass figure, hairstyles were *à la garçonne*, clothes were cut straight, hiding the body's curves, the figure was androgynous. Lipstick became the last, and almost only gender marker. And then the movement took off: in 1926, Jeanne Lanvin launched a lipstick in two versions, light and dark; at the beginning of the 1930s she had three colors, in 1938 six, in 1941 eight.

Meanwhile Elizabeth Arden was still recommending "a trace of color on your lips"; a trace indeed. "Make sure that your lip pencil matches your blusher. First the upper lip: two little strokes following the natural contours; then the lower lip. Make the paste penetrate gently. Nothing will spoil your appearance more quickly than badly made-up lips, and above all, don't use too much lipstick—just enough to emphasize your lips. Miss Arden has created a set of pencils: Chariot, Printemps, Victoire, Mat Victoire, Capucine, Coquette, Viola, Carmenita, and another exquisitely warm tone that goes particularly well with red hair, Red Head. The pencils are indelible."

At the dawn of World War II, Revlon was the first to match lipstick with nail enamel. In 1954, Dior

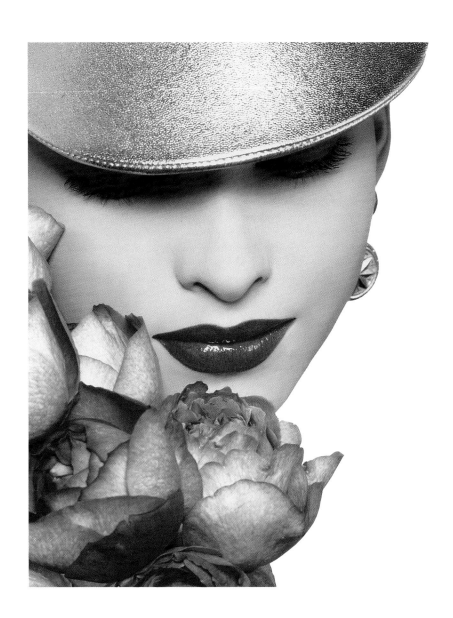

launched his lipstick as a substitute item of clothing, a color to wear, a way to dress the mouth, at least, in Dior if you couldn't afford anything else. The two new Hi-Fi colors by Max Factor in 1959 were called Shangri-la and Soleil Levant. Ranges continued to expand until MAC was offering 135 different colors of lipstick. In fall 1979, Dior's Chocs Clairs—three lipsticks and three nail enamels, gray, deep purple and beige—were an innovation for their creators, Serge Lutens and Annie Raynal, but met with a lukewarm reception everywhere except in the United States.

But in the space of a century, and throughout the world, the heart-shaped mouth had become the rainbow mouth.

Effets de Fleurs, a transparent lipstick by Dior, summer 1995. Photograph by Tyen. Preceding pages: Mixtures for pearly-finish lipsticks ("cloisonné orange and satin red") at the Parfums Dior factory (left), and By Terry lipsticks (right).

Pure Color, Estée Lauder's
latest lipstick (below)
and Color Gloss, the new
Rouge Absolu colors by
Lancôme (left).
Right: This mouth is unique!
Advertisement for Manifesto,
the new line of make-up
created by Isabella Rossellini
for Lancaster: style and
individuality first!

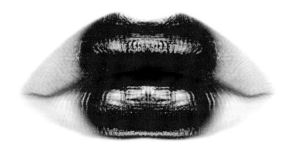

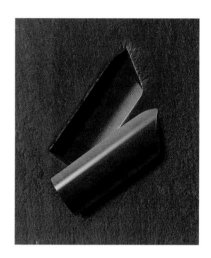

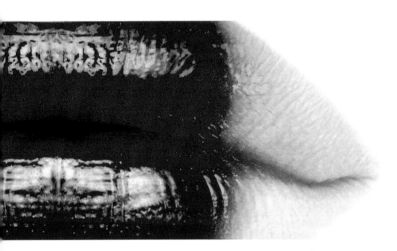

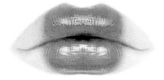

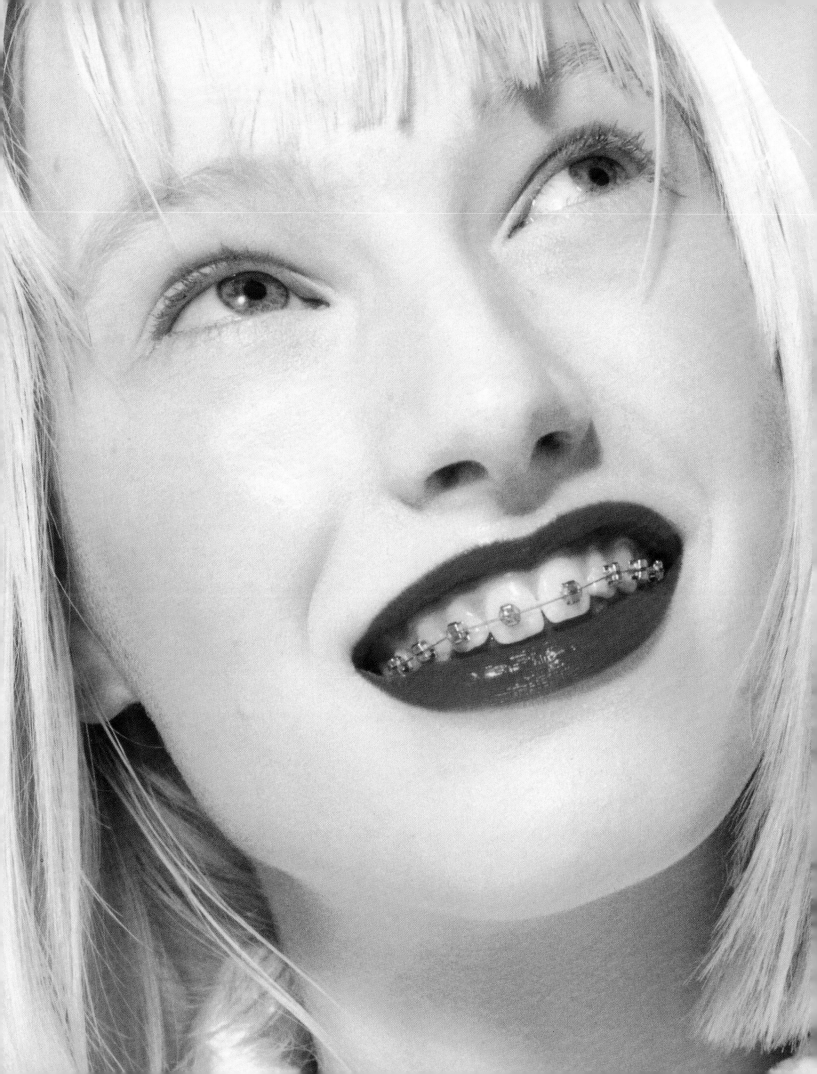

Right down to the...

fingertips

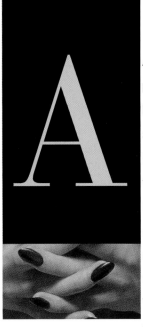

After the punks and their safety-pins, fashion continued in rather brutal vein with piercing, but skin decoration now seems to have come back to the surface, with more reversible practices. Make-up has always been ephemeral by nature . . . and drawing and collage can now be used in addition to painting. We can tattoo pictures onto our skin, or decorate it with glitter, transfers, beauty spots and other "ready-mades"—echoes of twentieth-century art. We may describe this superficial, throw-away kind of make-up as "morphing," but in fact it is merely a logical extension of traditional make-up, which can now be applied to other parts of the body. Our hair can now be "made up" too, with products that wash out with the first shampoo, as opposed to permanent dyes.

"Does not fashion govern kings themselves?"
Memoirs of Baroness d'Oberkirch

Sisters under the Skin,
by Norman Parkinson,
1978.

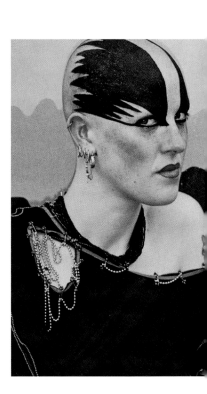

Right: Dalí painting sun-ray wrinkles on Gala's forehead.
Previous page:
Shiseido polishes, 1973.

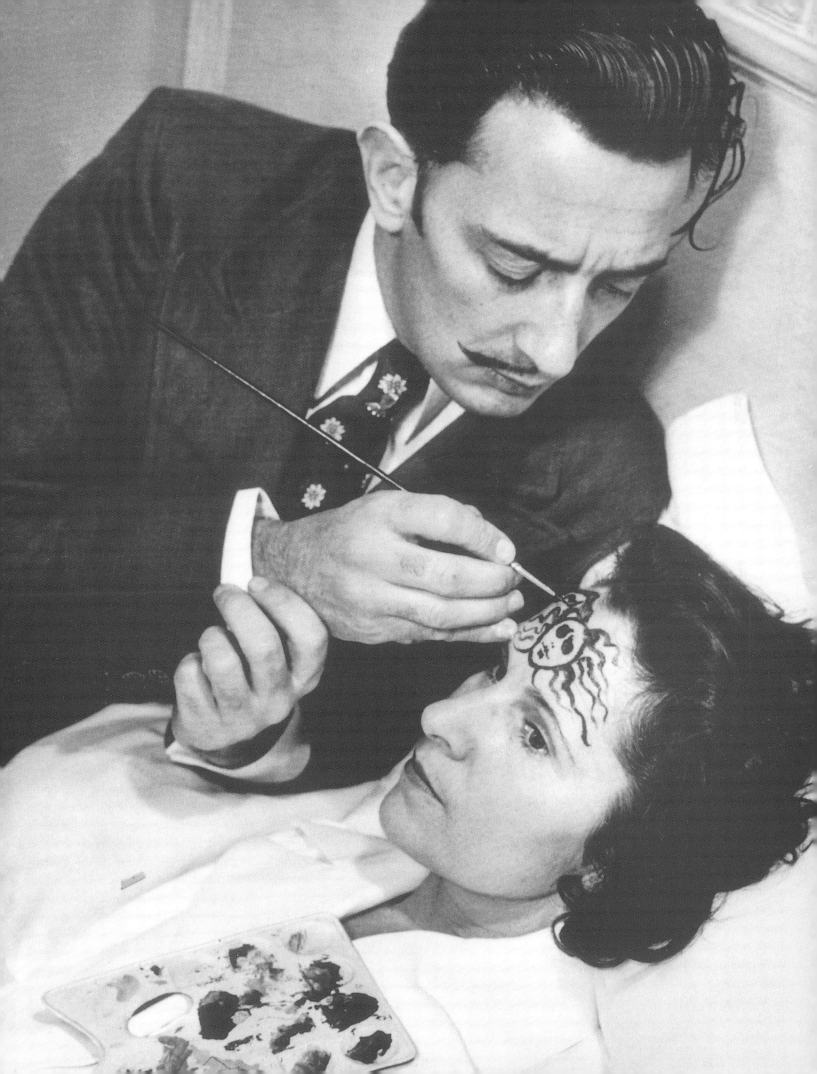

1
6
2

A box for beauty-spot patches, trimmed with pearls and flowering branches in pink and green gold, ca. 1780; Musée des Arts Décoratifs, Paris. Below: Marisa Berenson and Ryan O'Neal in Stanley Kubrick's *Barry Lyndon*, 1975, a film rich in pictorial references, from Chardin to Gainsborough.

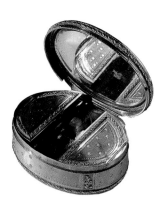

In the spring of 1646, the French comic dramatist Paul Scarron wrote to Mme d'Hautefort of the fashion in Le Mans: "Glitter now adorns the face / That beauty spots were wont to grace."

And glitter is back! In 1995, Jeanne Moreau was all aglow with it, for the presentation of the César awards. During the same period, at Dior, Annie Raynal created products containing glitter that spangled with a whole range of colors. Yves Rocher cosmetics now include stick-on pearls, and Lancôme has "Crystal teardrops": drops of Swarovski crystal to place at the corner of the eye, or in the cleavage. And not long ago, Bourjois relaunched the beauty spot.

Deciphering the beauty spot

Beauty spot patches appeared during the reign of Henri IV. For a time they were worn by men—even by the gallant court clergy—then they became a feminine preserve once again.

These patches were of various shapes and sizes, and were positioned differently according to the time of day and the occasion. The result formed a kind of secret code. For the "précieuses"—whom Mme de Sévigné called "the dears"—each patch had a name and a symbolic meaning in their games of amorous intrigue. A patch in the corner of the eye meant "passionate" or "provocative"; in the middle of the forehead, it was "majestic"; on the nose it meant "shameless" or "bold"; on the edge of a dimple in the cheek it was "cheerful"; on a pimple, "thieving." This beauty-spot language was long forgotten . . . but Fabrice Luchini brought it back to life in a famous seduction scene from a recent film by Christian Vincent, *La Discrète*.

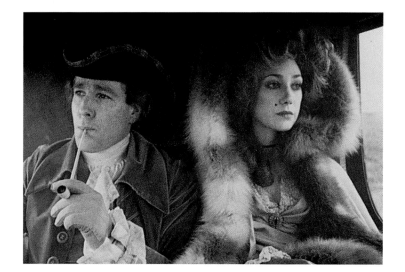

Right: Pietro Longhi's *Woman with a Beauty Spot*. Longhi wittily recorded Venetian life in his paintings, as Goldoni did in his plays.

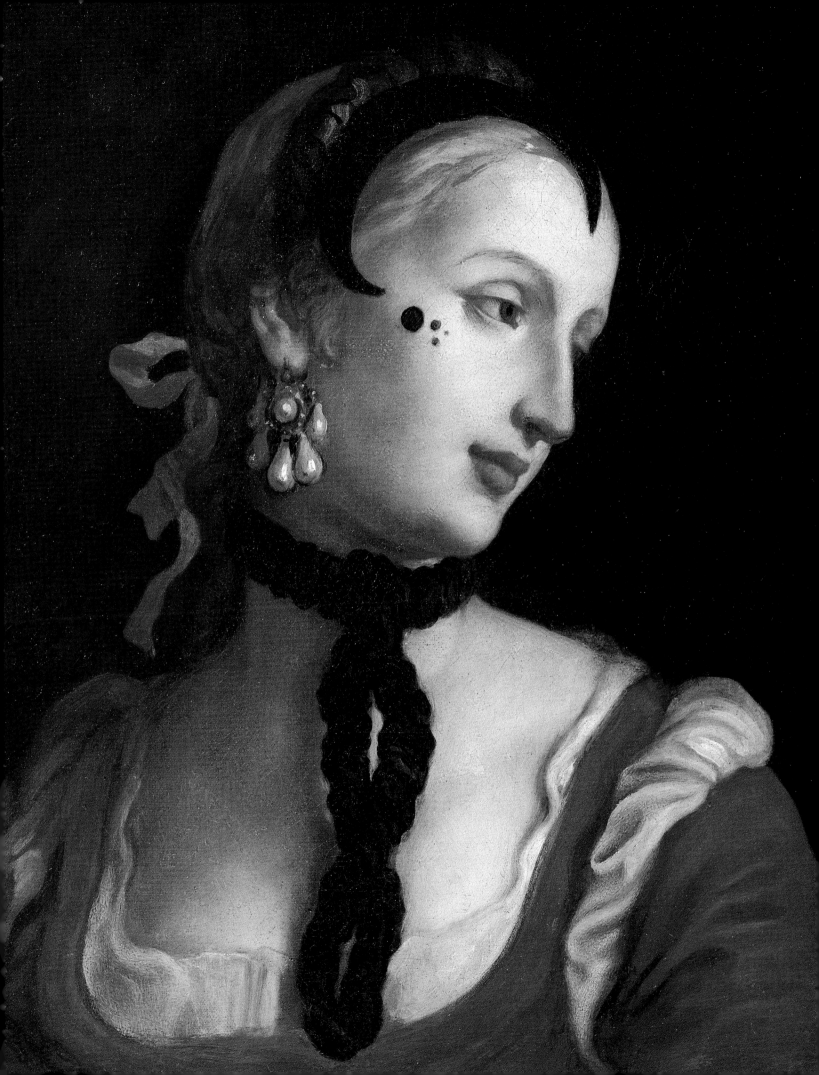

1
6
4

Stick-on taffeta patches were cut out in the shape of suns, moons, crescents, hearts, little characters and animals. In 1692, they could all be found in Paris, in a shop called A la Perle des Mouches, in the Rue Saint-Denis. During the reign of Louis XV, the fashion was for a large, black velvet patch, embellished with brilliants. Long before Braque and Picasso, the techniques of collage were already being used in the art of make-up.

As usual, a medical origin was found for this artifice. A toothache was treated at the time by placing tiny bandages, covered in taffeta or velvet, on the temples; the fashion-conscious realized that these discs enhanced the complexion—and a new fashion was launched. Louis Guyon was probably the first to suggest this explanation, in his *Diverses Leçons* (1625). Alfred Franklin found it there, and it has been widely repeated ever since. Yet it might be simpler to look for the origin of the patch elsewhere: it had always been used in China, and the European patch may just have been an imitation of an oriental original.

In the early second century A.D. (during the dynasty of the later Han), the poet Tchang Heng spoke of: "A chignon of jet-black hair / Shiny enough to be used as a mirror / And a patch to enhance her engaging smile." Chinese women had already been wearing patches for over a century; they put them at the corner of their mouths or on their foreheads. The most popular were called *hoa-tze* ("flowers"); these were little round discs cut out of black paper. There were also more decorative patches, in five different colors.

One of the "speckled" wood and stone statuettes of the Tang dynasty (seventh–ninth centuries).

Chinese women often wore a larger beauty spot on their foreheads too; it was crescent-shaped, painted in yellow ointment, and was called "patch of the yellow star" or "yellow mark between the eyebrows." This fashion lasted well into the Ming period. It only fell into disuse during the Manchu dynasty, which ruled China from 1644.

Naturally, the Chinese also found a utilitarian explanation for patches. According to a Tang author, the patch was originally used to conceal marks made by a hot iron; he maintained that vindictive wives used to brand concubines' faces out of jealousy . . . or to punish them for some offence.

It seems highly unlikely, however, that a branding iron would leave marks so small that a patch could cover them . . . creams or powders would surely have been more useful. No, the only explanation for these cosmetic practices is a symbolic one. And if patches have a secret language, let's try to understand what powder has to say!

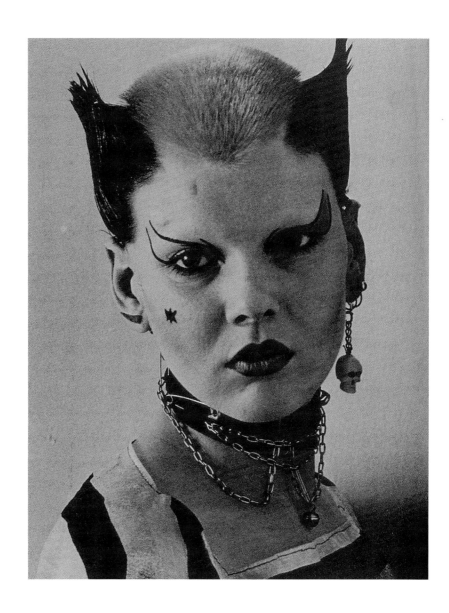

Mephistophelean
punkette,
England, 1980s.

Right down to the . . . fingertips

The power of powder

When Charles Trénet sang "We put cosmetics in our hair" (*Fleur Bleue,* 1937), he was referring to a sticky lotion like Brylcreem, the sort of preparation used by Spanish tango-dancers. Before the days of brilliantine, powder had been widely used. Hair powder dates back to earliest antiquity; but it was not much used in France before Charles IX. During the reign of Henri III, red or yellowish powder was in constant use. In 1577, Venetian ambassadors reported that "the king has had all his hair shaved off, on his doctor's advice. He wears a very splendid and beautiful postiche, covered in musky violet powder." Following the example of the king and his extravagant minions, all and sundry wanted to be covered in powder, and the clergy raged—in vain—against women who appeared in holy places "powdered like millers."

From the French Regency (of the Duke of Orleans, from 1715 to 1723) onward, hair was either lightly frosted or buried under an avalanche of powder! Silver was held to be the most elegant color at the time, but all sorts of colors were produced. Poor women made their hair-powder from bits of rotten wood—again according to Louis Guyon—but the nobility made theirs from a perfumed mixture of wheat flours and beans.

This extraordinary fashion lasted until the Revolution, scandalizing the less frivolous members of the population. They claimed that the quantities of flour thus transformed into powder were enough to provide daily food for ten thousand poor peasants—as the historian Mercier relates in his *Tableau de Paris*— or that as much flour went onto an aristocrat's head as into his stomach. Their figures may have been exaggerated, but there is no doubt that it was an exceptionally wasteful practice.

The powdering process itself took place amid a dense cloud that

An interpretation of an eighteenth-century hairstyle: Tina Aumont in Fellini's *Casanova*, 1976.
Right: Valentino Moon, another Fellinian actor, with plastered-down hair and darkened eyes.

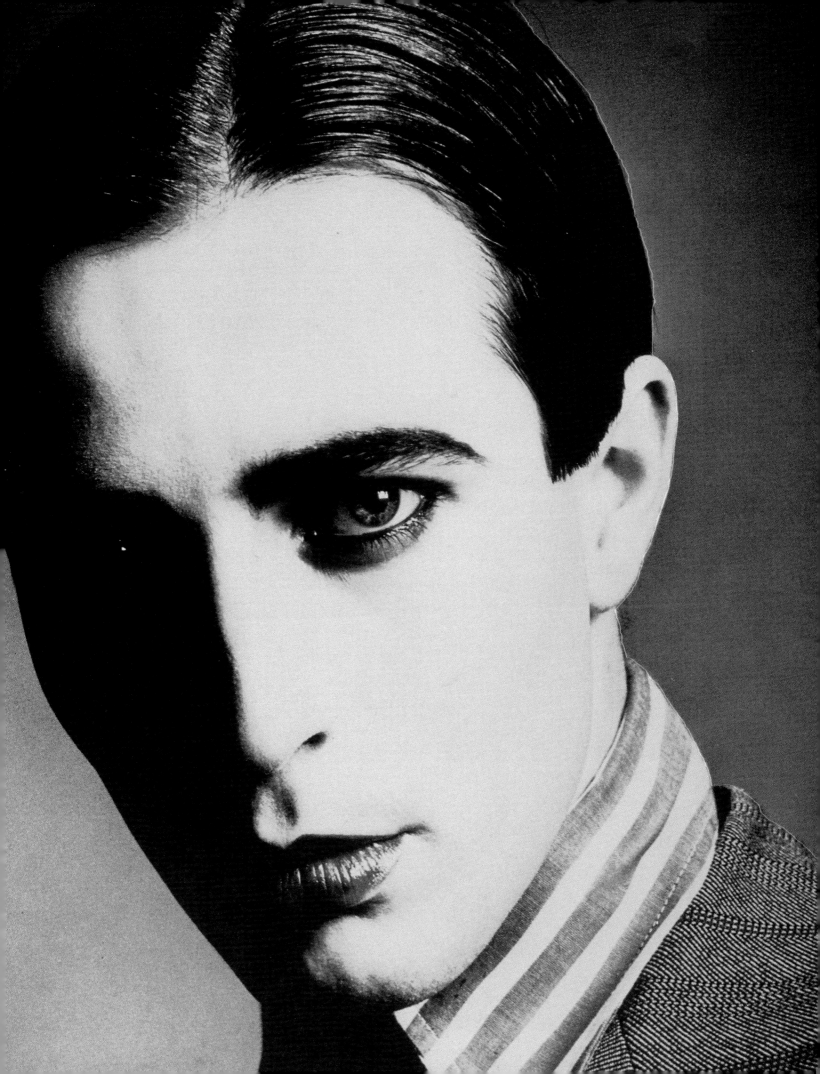

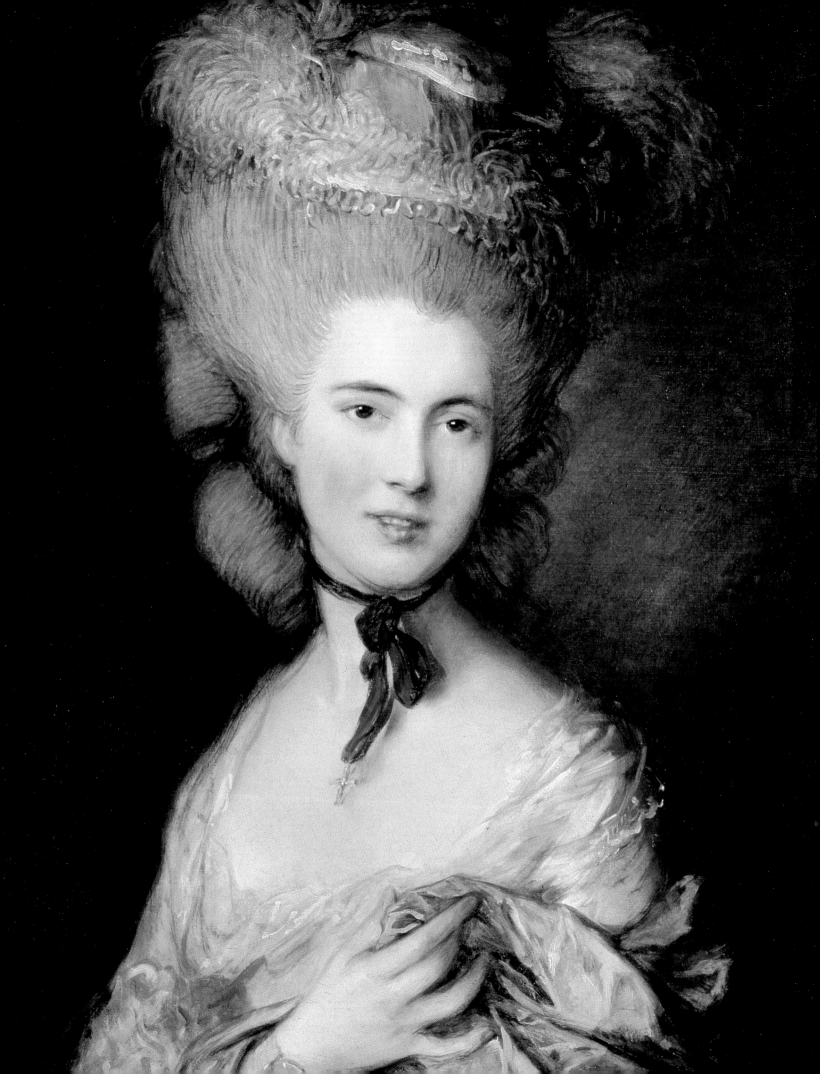

the hairdresser created around the client, who was wrapped up in a huge dressing gown, with his head in a conical paper nosebag to avoid suffocation! The hairdressers themselves emerged floured like fish ready for the frying pan, which is why they were nicknamed "whitings": "Then we see wigmaker-boys, commonly known as whitings because they are floured from head to toe; you must avoid them if you are wearing black, because they will make you white and greasy," said Mercier.

So much for the picturesque aspect. But maybe the aristocracy was making a last, desperate gesture by throwing all this flour so liberally around . . . they were, in fact, ostentatiously squandering the very source of their wealth, the income they received in kind from their lands. Perhaps the flour in which they were drowning reminded them of their bygone power, rooted in rural fiefs? It was said that the provincial nobles had come to court "bearing their meadows and mills on their shoulders." At Versailles, they were enslaved and subjugated, and they wept for their lost independence, the dusty paths of adventure, the age when vassal was not yet synonymous with valet.

Finally, for the court of the Sun King on the eve of the Revolution, all this powder may have symbolized the powder of the battlefield . . . and, sensing that this was a battle they were bound to lose, they were celebrating their own funeral by covering their heads with ashes.

Smallpox and bigwigs!

Nowadays we are more playful. We put mascara or glitter in our hair, or apply colorful arabesques with an inking-pad . . . and sometimes they even glow in the dark! The tradition of hair adornment goes back a long way: people have put just about everything in their hair . . . even the garden gnome would have found his way there if he weren't so heavy!

The Baroness d'Oberkirch tells the following anecdote: "Mourning for the King [Louis XV] put a stop for a while to a rather ridiculous new fashion which replaced the quèsaco [the feathered bonnets called Panaches de Quèsaco, launched by Mlle Bertin in 1771]: the *poufs au sentiment*. This was a hairstyle, into which one put one's favorite people or things. So in went the portrait of one's daughter or mother, the picture of one's canary, or dog, etc., together with a lock of hair from the head of one's father or

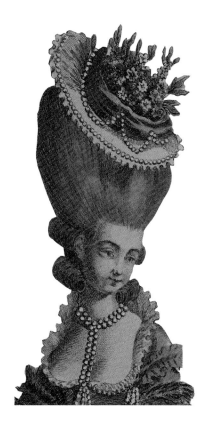

Marie-Antoinette hairstyle, a good century before the Eiffel Tower!
Left: *Portrait of the Duchess of Beaufort*, ca. 1780, by Gainsborough (who had a hat named after him: the one that the Duchess of Devonshire was wearing in the portrait he painted of her).

"Put sunflower seeds
in a woman's breast milk . . .
Extract the oil, and heat
gold leaf in it . . . plaster your
hair with it, and it will look like
the finest gold." According
to Giovanni Marinello, anyway!
Below: Hair tattoo by Tyen,
for Dior, summer 1999.

1
7
0

Right down to the . . . fingertips

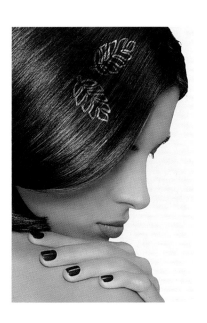

sweetheart. It was incredibly extravagant. We nevertheless wanted to conform to it, and the mischievous princess [Dorothy de Württemberg, fourteen years old] wore on her ear, all day long, the figure of a woman holding a bunch of keys, whom she insisted was Madame Hendel [the housekeeper at Montbéliard castle]. The latter found it a remarkable likeness, and nearly died of joy and pride."

Even more comical were the *poufs au sentiment* on the theme of the cow-pox inoculation—Jenner's vaccination against smallpox, which had its enthusiasts among the most highly placed at court.

Such extravagance! And yet we have only mentioned the things people put in their hair, not the way they styled it. Hair fashion soon became a very tyrannical business. Hairdressers were well aware that they were creating a look both for immediate effect, and one to be admired for centuries to come:

"Painters and sculptors often portray the woman once she has been styled by our care," wrote the hairdressers' lawyer, in an attempt to dissuade Louis XVI from including "ladies' hairdressers" in the guild of "barbers, wigmakers, bathers and steamers."

There were already heated arguments as to whether one should follow the fashion or develop a personal style. Carlo Goldoni, who disliked "disheveled hair, with locks hanging over the eyebrows, [which] give [women] disadvantages they would do better to avoid," advised: "Women are wrong to follow the general fashion as regards their hair, whose styling is so essential to enhance their grace and beauty; each woman should consult her mirror, examine her features, adapt the arrangement of her hair to the appearance of her face, and guide the hand of her wigmaker."

All over the world and all through history, the art of hairdressing has produced the most amazing constructions, and hair itself has undergone a great many processes to modify its color. Aztec women, to take just one of many possible examples, wove feathers into their hair, which they dyed a variety of colors. However, only Venetian-style bleaching corresponds to our definition of make-up as being essentially ephemeral. Rodocanachi wrote: "Most Italian women 'washed their hair,' as they said [this was around 1600], at least twice a week, and after each operation, their hair acquired that magnificent blond tone with tawny highlights which was the glory, albeit usurped, of Venetian women. Now [around 1700] this habit is dying out, and black hair is coming back, except among those women who traffic their charms."

Almost all courtesans were blond; and the distinctive signs they were ordered by law to wear on their clothing were usually yellow too.

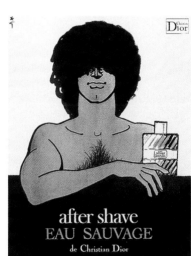

A Gruau poster for the Dior aftershave Eau Sauvage, 1972.

In 1758, the 17,000 soldiers of Charles-Eugène de Württemberg's army sported 17,000 mustaches, which had to be black, whatever the color of the hair. If a man's mustache was not thick enough or did not correspond to the norms in some way, he had to wear a false one.

"His beard and mustache used to be a man's make-up," wrote L-A de Caraccioli. They could be brilliantined and sometimes dyed, but black was the rule, and anything else was considered effeminate: "A big mustache and a fringe of hair over the forehead, dyed peroxide blond" went with "a heavily made-up face, mascara on the eyelashes, rouged cheeks . . ." (J. Lorrain).

These days, rugby and soccer players appear on television with bright blond streaks in their hair. The range of cosmetics for men now includes tanning powders (Guerlain for example), but there is nothing feminine about the approach: "Terracotta for men is different: its color is a muted copper; its aspect is matte, without iridescence; its presentation is original, and as virile as a shaving bowl held firmly in the hand."

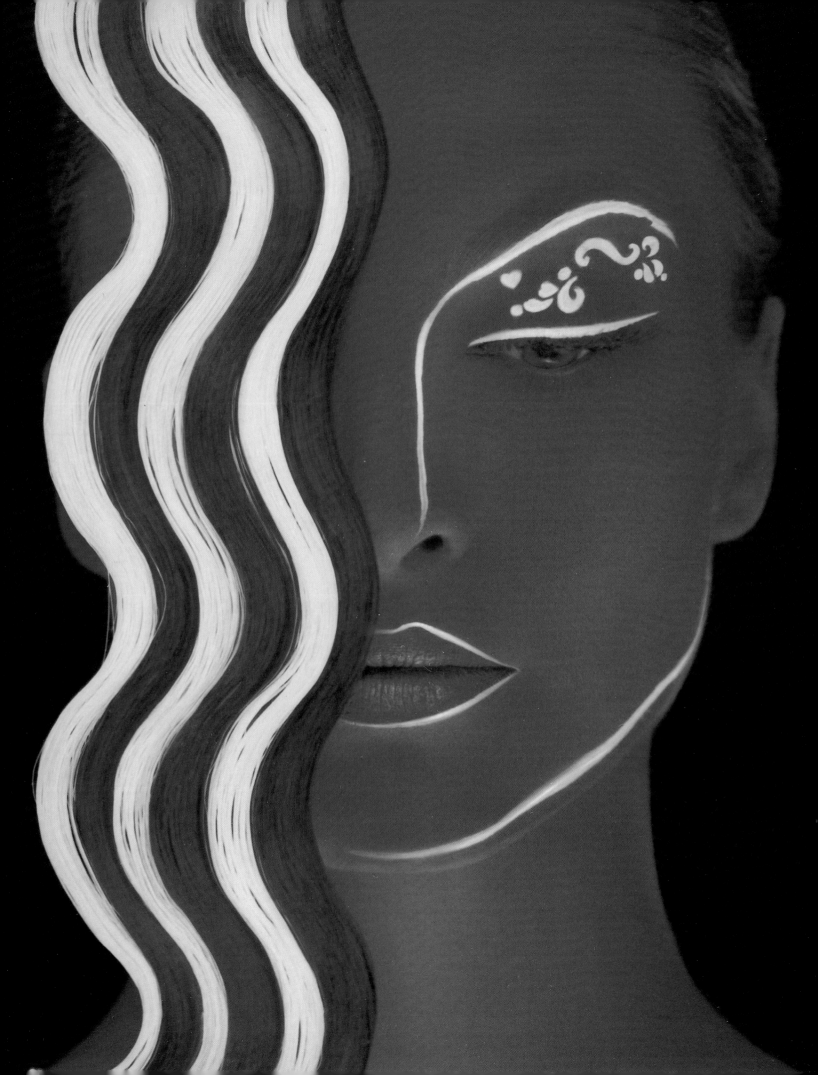

Mascara flash (below) and Dior's Lumière Noire range (left), by Tyen, director of Make-up and Beauty Creation, who brought his talent for harmony from the opera to the world of cosmetics.

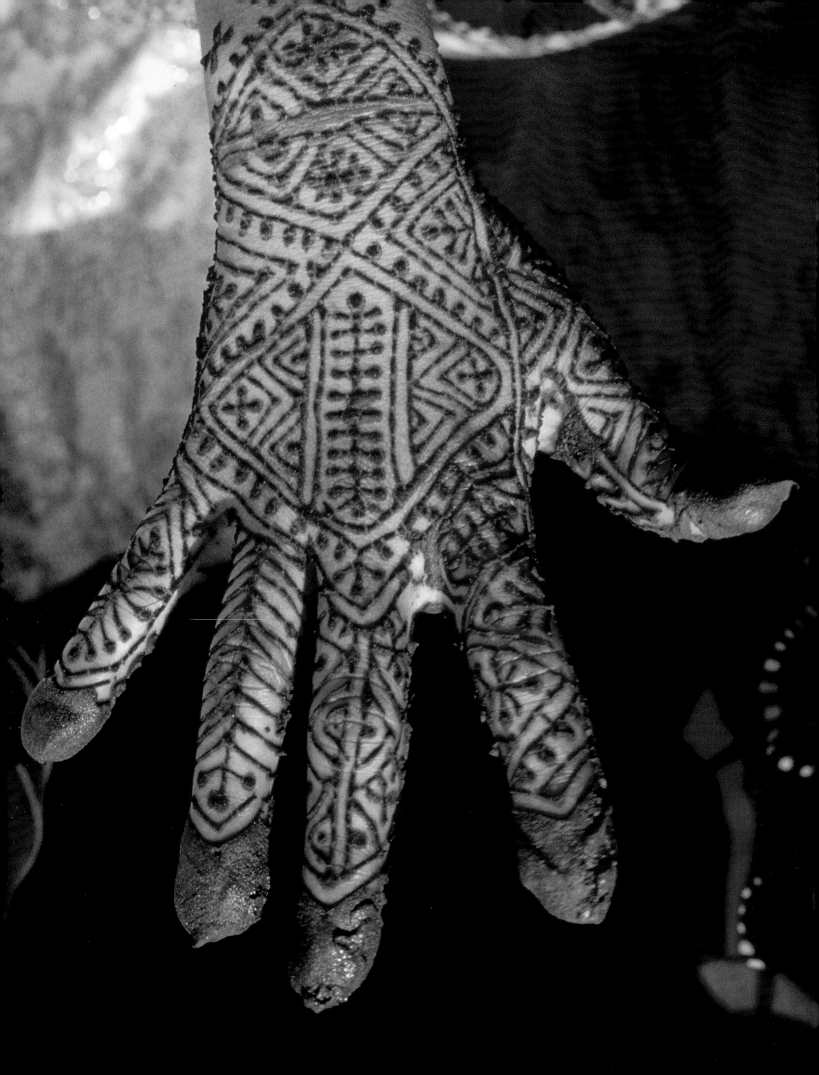

Exotic cosmetics

Yellow is now just another element in the make-up kaleidoscope, so let's take another look at the more classical colors. According to Haafner: "Instead of wearing patches on their faces as European women used to, Indian dancers wear blue marks. They paint the tips of their fingernails with red dye extracted from a plant called mindie or lakscha.

"In Bengal, women put similar marks on their faces, but also on their arms and other parts of the body, except the throat. Sometimes they even use the tip of a needle to draw figures of all kinds, into which they rub fine charcoal or gunpowder."

Today's tattoos have no military connotation! In 1988, Bourjois launched their Tattoos—simple inking-pads—and 600,000 were sold! They come in three colors, one of which is royal henna. The same brand also has a Skin Jewelry range: adhesive stencils that you fill in with eye-liner. The novelty of products like these is their painless application; but they are still worn on the traditional spots where ethnologists, like Marcel Mauss, have always seen them. "Most tattoos are put on parts of the body where you can see the pulse: on the ankles, the wrists or the neck."

The Mendhi kits, by l'Oréal, include stencils and a fine brush for painting with henna; and the Trompe-l'œil consists of henna motifs, which are not applied directly onto the skin, but onto transparent plastic film which can then be worn as rings, bracelets, necklaces or belts.

In Islamic countries, henna is used to color hands, nails, arms and heels. "The leaves of the *Lawsonia inermis* are dried and reduced to a greenish powder," explains Eugène Rimmel, member of the London Society of Arts and the horticultural societies of London and Nice. "A little water is added to make a paste, which is applied to the skin and wrapped in strips of cloth; after two or three hours, a reddish-yellow color is produced, which will withstand repeated washings."

In Turkey, this dye is only used on the nails, where henna leaves a brighter, longer-lasting color than on the skin. In Egypt, it is used on the

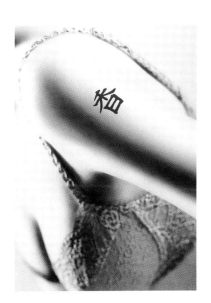

Body Tattoo, by Bourjois: tattooing without pain. Left: The hennaed hand of a future bride. Marrakech, Morocco, 1990s.

finger- and toenails, but also on the palms of the hand, the soles of the feet, and the fingers up to the first phalanx. Some fashion-conscious women dye a band on their second or third phalanx, and little circles on their knuckles. Bandages are left on overnight, and the application is renewed every two or three weeks. Finally, some add a mixture of lampblack, lime and linseed oil to the hennaed places, which makes them a beautiful ebony color, and they alternate red and black from one phalanx to another. Henna may be applied in symbolic motifs and is sometimes thought to bring good luck.

According to Lane: "In rural areas, women of the lower classes tattoo—at the very least—their chin and the back of their right hand, and lower-class urban women do the same, to a lesser extent. They prick the skin with seven needles, then rub in a mixture of lampblack and woman's breast milk; about a week later, they rub in a paste made of fresh beetroot leaves and clover, which leaves a blue or greenish color—or they can apply indigo straight away if they want to speed up the process."

In Japan, during the nineteenth century, the fashion for tattooing was developed as an art form, called *horimono*. The people of Edo (later called Tokyo) and many courtesans went to tattooers, who usually found the inspiration for their work in legendary themes or kabuki. This art died out during the twentieth century, surviving only among geishas and actors.

Claude Lévi-Strauss, who observed the Kaduveo Indians of southern Brazil, reported that the art of tattooing was an exclusively female domain: "They lived naked, and spent their days covering each other's bodies and faces with a network of painted arabesques, of unforgettable delicacy and elegance."

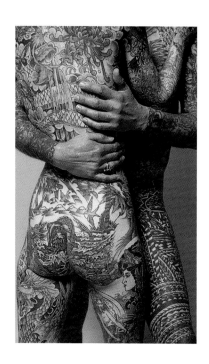

Horimono, the art of tattooing which was back in fashion in the nineteenth century, gained followers in the West: a tattooed couple in the United States in 1984 (left). Right: Jean-Paul Gaultier model, 1994.

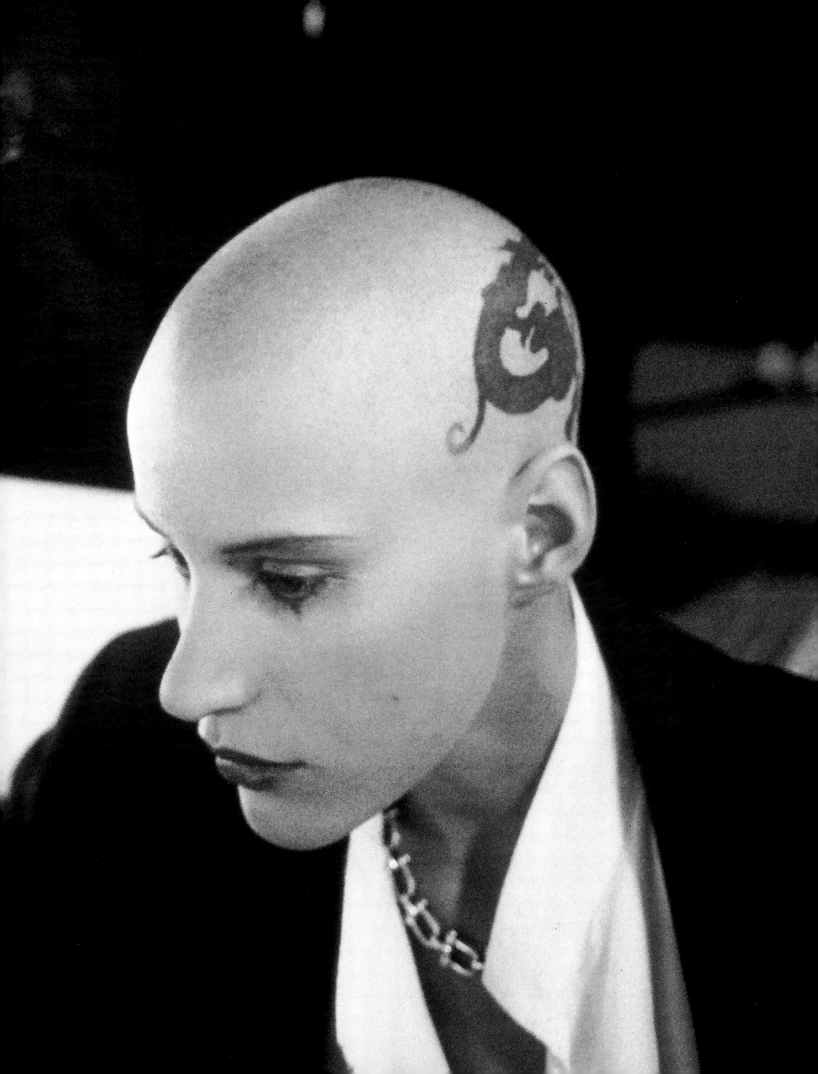

Young Kayapo Indians of
present-day Brazil.
The purest vegetable red
makes a splendid make-up,
for festivities which last
a whole day.

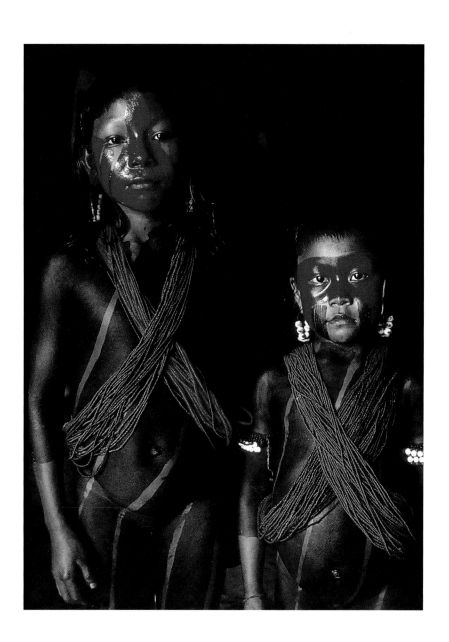

In the northwest of the Amazon region, make-up is virtually the only tradition left to the Yawanawas, who have neither feathered headdresses, nor sculpted artifacts, nor musical instruments; it is in fact their only art form. They make themselves up for festivals—or *mariri*—but also for no particular reason. They pierce the fresh fruit of the urucum with a little stick, and paint its red directly onto their bodies—it all disappears at the first wash. They also use a black coloring, jenipapo, which darkens in the open air, and lasts nearly a month.

The fruit of the urucum, or annatto tree, forms a conical capsule covered in thorns. The seeds of the same fruit are also used to make a paste—annatto—of a pale salmon, orangy color, which is used as a food coloring. The Yawanawas owe their survival to the latex from their native hevea: when the rubber market collapsed, the American cosmetics firm Aveda planted 23,000 urucum for them, made them the gift of a military hospital from the Vietnam war, and made them the mascots of their ecological lipstick . . . But it continues to buy the output produced from classic plantations, which are closer to less expensive means of transport.

In recent haute-couture fashion shows, we have seen models with motifs painted down their legs. During World War II, many ersatz products were created, like seamed stockings painted onto the skin, and suitably inventive products were sold by cosmeticians. "Thanks to Elizabeth Arden, who thinks of everything," wrote the *Œuvre* on May 20, 1941, "we can veil our legs decently, with no fear of snagging. The artificial silk stocking is born; no other stocking is as reliable." This marvel cost 35 francs; and, for 30 francs, René Rambaud proposed the "seamless stocking" in a range of three colors: flesh, gold and tan. Filpas, by the perfumer Bienaimé, cost 24 francs a bottle: "Silk on your legs without stockings. It isn't a dye . . . but it covers the skin and sheathes the legs like the prettiest of stockings."

Haute Couture collection 1999–2000, by John Galliano for Christian Dior. A far cry from the traditional pink and gray of the family house in Granville . . .

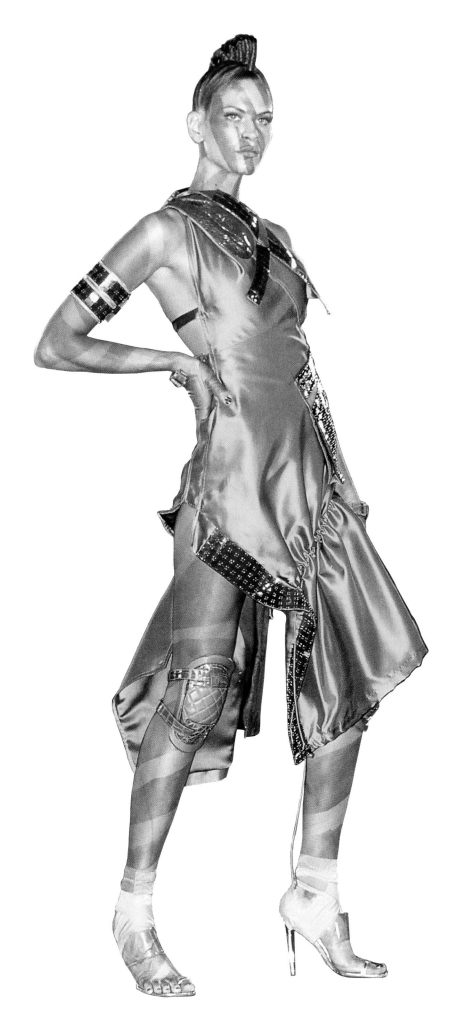

Right down to the . . . fingertips

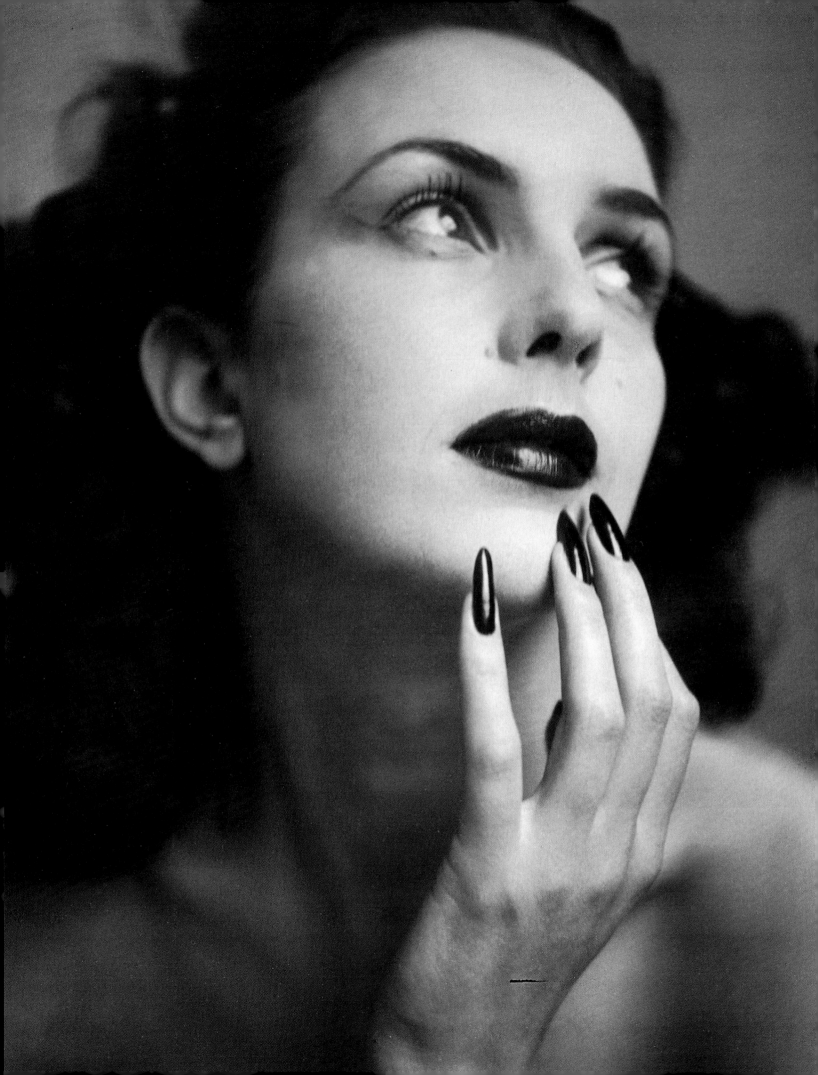

Finishing touches

All kinds of painting need varnish: it adds the finishing touch to any work of art, be it performed on the easel or on the body. A work of make-up should go from top to toe—finger and toenails included! Varnish and lacquer are exotic products, originating in the Far East; in Changsha, in the southern province of Hunan, inside a tomb from the fourth or third centuries B.C., enameled boxes, beauty kits and lacquered mirrors were found. This region remained the center for "Coromandel" lacquers, so-called because they were dispatched from the Coromandel Coast by the East India Company.

China and Japan may both claim to have been the first to use lacquer, but the American firm Revlon claims to have invented opaque nail enamel in 1932, to replace transparent polish; they started using pigments rather than dyes to create a wide range of pinks, corals, and reds. But colors, like fashions, change cyclically, and in the early 1960s colorless enamels were back. In 1962, nail enamels were part of the Dior color explosion. In 1977, a daring navy blue (Boubou Blue) was launched to wear with jeans, and a lovely green was also created. Today, we can buy pastel or acid tones from Hard Candy; Urban Decay (who had already launched Drag Queen) has polishes the color of Smarties, and picturesque tones like rust and dust from the streets of Manhattan; and Guerlain has a Belle de Nuit enamel, which is discreetly golden in the light of day and becomes phosphorescent in black light. And, to encourage anyone who still can't be bothered to put it on . . . the incomparable lacquer of the land of the rising sun requires thirty coats! Each one is applied with a fine hair brush, and buffed with charcoal; and the final coat is polished with ash from a doe's horn.

In the fifth century B.C., in Delphi and in Athens, the range of colors for painting had progressed from monochrome to four colors: white, yellow, red and black. The Ancients only ever used those four. Around 1500, in Venice, the great colorist Giorgione was still using the same four colors: "He painted all flesh

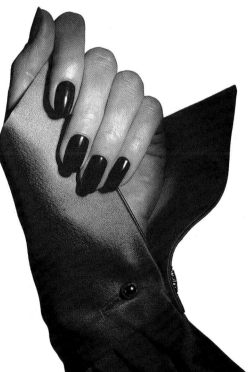

"Tentation", by Dior. The nail enamel for spring 1992, by Tyen.

Left: Beautiful to the tips of her fingers . . . Florette, as always, photographed by J.-H. Lartigue in 1943.

Clark Gable smiles
his seductive smile at the
*Naked Woman at her
Dressing Table*,
photographed by
Paul Outerbridge in 1936.

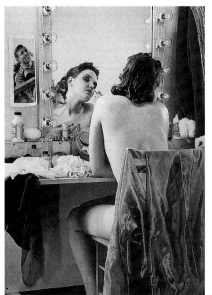

tints with them, whatever the age
and sex," said Diderot.

Make-up remained classical
longer than painting, with red, white
and black for the face, plus yellow in
Asia, and hair color in the West. If,
as Maurice Denis said, all painting
"is essentially a flat surface, covered
in colors assembled in a certain
order . . ." then it's easy! When the
explosion of colors finally took place,
it was just a question of putting
them on properly!

Basically, from whatever angle
one approaches the subject of
make-up, from the roots of the hair
to the tips of the toes, the objective
is the same: to please. Make-up to
please others, or to please oneself.
Make-up to put on a good show, for
nobody in particular and for the

world in general. Make-up to create
an illusion, for theater audiences or
TV viewers. Make-up to celebrate a
cult: to please the gods, to worship
or appease them. Make-up as a
corrector of the ravages of time: to
keep on pleasing.

And if we cross to the other side
of the looking glass, to look at things
from the manufacturer's point of
view, the aim is still to please—but
this time it's to please the consumer
and to sell the product.

The point is to get oneself
noticed, rather than play the
wallflower or fade into the
background—to state one's
individuality, in whatever color or
tone one chooses.

Throughout the ages, the means
to achieve this goal have varied.

Cary Grant succumbs
to the charms of
Katharine Hepburn in
Howard Hawks's film
Bringing up Baby, 1938.

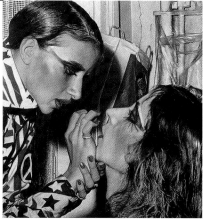

Despite appearances,
the hairdresser is a woman
and the model is a man.
Marina and Luciano,
by Franz Gertsch, 1975.

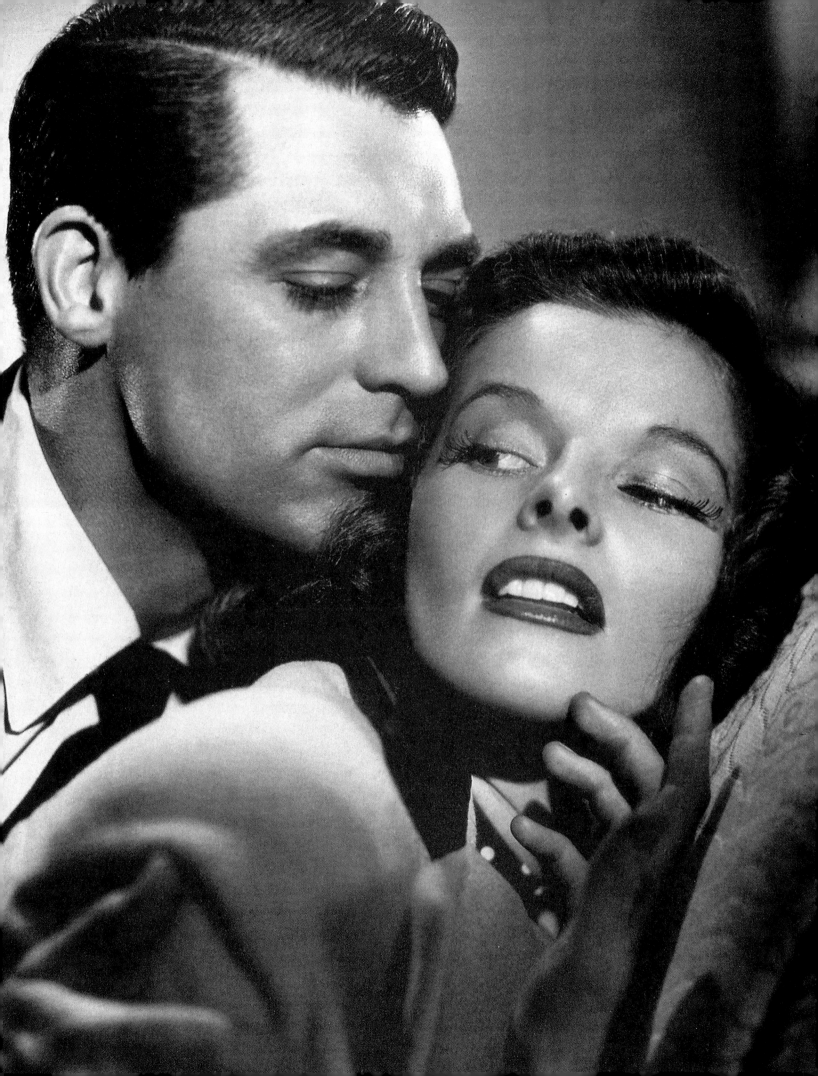

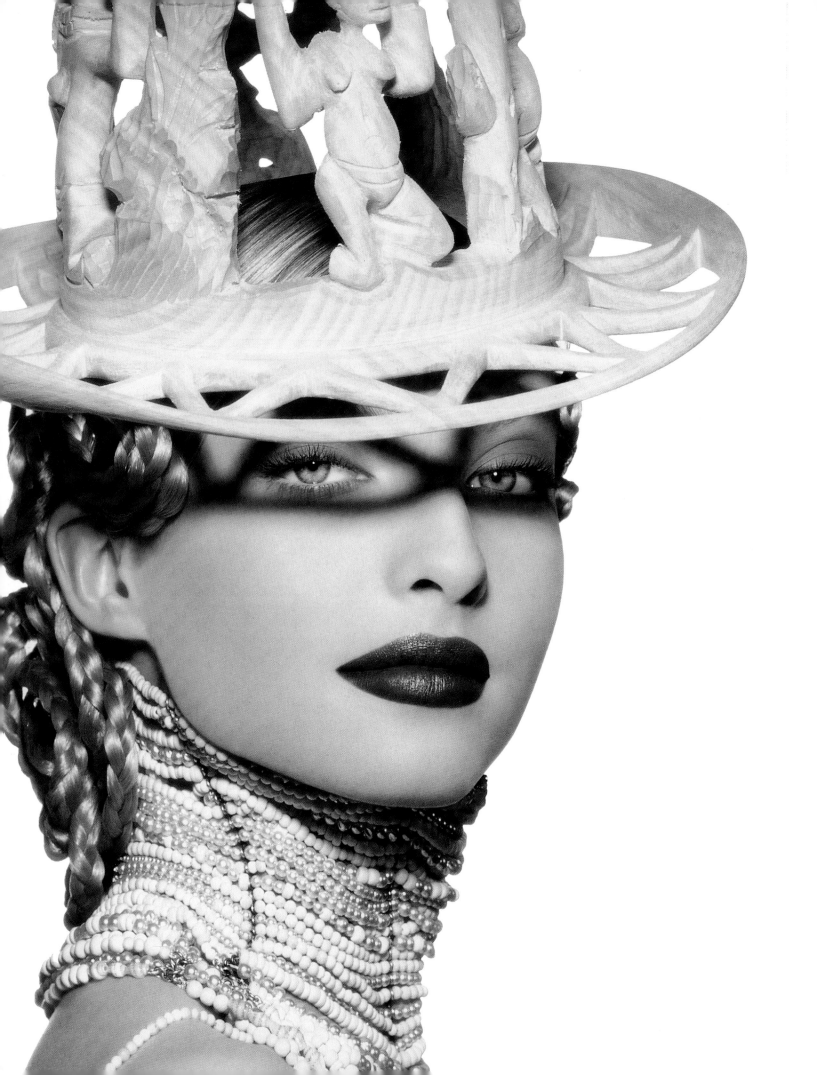

Sometimes the emphasis is on the beauty of the end product, like a painting. The aesthetic pleasure of wearing beautiful cosmetic products is similar to that of wearing precious jewelry. At other times, make-up is used to underline one's difference, to emphasize one's originality—green eyes, full lips . . . This second approach might seem paradoxical: to "make up," after all, means to imagine, to invent—and to deceive, as it's a superficial art which hides the reality underneath. Yet nowadays the idea is to "reveal" or "express" oneself.

Scientific progress has resulted in "see-through" colors, a miraculous combination of density and translucence—perhaps symbolizing the myth of transparence in a society where communication is everywhere—but only skin deep.

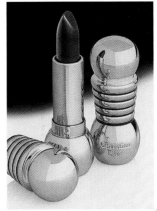

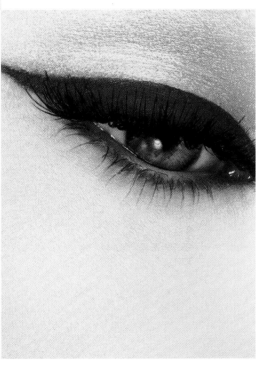

Diorific lipstick (top)
and Duoliner double eyeliner
(above).
Left: Christian Dior. Wooden
hat from the John Galliano
collection and giraffe-woman
necklace, to go with
the Diorific look by Tyen.

"Fashions come and go,

placing the emphasis

on different parts of the body,

thereby shifting attention

and renewing attraction.

It is interesting to see that

the criteria for charm

vary from one generation

to the next—but that there are

relative constants within

the same generation"

Christian Dior

Glossary

Blush: A dry make-up; the word first appeared in the 1960s, probably 1969.

Cake: A synonym for compact powder. Pancake is in a flat shape; panstick is like lipstick.

Eyeliner: A dark liquid make-up used to emphasize the eyebrows or eyelids.

Foundation: Obviously, the base for everything; it first appeared around 1910.

Gloss: A synonym for sheen, slick.

Kohl: Also spelled khôl, kohol, kohel. The spelling doesn't really matter unless you're playing scrabble. The word comes from a seventeenth-century Arabic word for eye make-up.

Mascara: Eyelash make-up that first appeared in 1922.

Powder: The expression first appeared in 1845 in a reference to rice powder. Today powder is either compact or loose.

Rimmel: A patented name for eye make-up, in common use since 1929.

Rouge: This word has designated a certain kind of make-up since 1690.

Short history of brand names

Elizabeth Arden

No such person ever existed; this name was created—and slightly altered—from the first and last words of a successful book title: *Elizabeth and her German Garden*. The company began in 1910 with a beauty parlor on New York's Fifth Avenue, followed by another one on Place Vendôme in Paris in 1921. The initial products were beauty treatments. It is now owned by the Unilever group.

Bourjois

This company first appeared in 1863 with theater products, and Sarah Bernhardt was their most famous client. Ready-to-use make-up, but of a sort used on the stage. Rouge, rice powder and the first compact powder then become more common with everyday women, just before the Roaring Twenties.

Caron

This was not Auguste Caron, the model for Balzac's César Birotteau, but a company founded in 1904. Peau Fine, one of the first compact powders, was extremely successful prior to World War I. Today Caron is part of the Cora-Revillon group.

Chanel

Although beauty products and make-up were sold as early as the 1920s, Beauté Chanel was created in 1975, with several new ideas: it started to sell Coco's favorite rouge, and launched Édition Ephémère, products that were sold for a single season only.

Dior

This is the Haute-Couture of rouge and powders. In 1954, New Look was launched for lips; by 1969, Dior had expanded to an entire line, from foundation to nail enamel. The following year, specific make-up ranges were created for each season. Each season range is called "look" and has its specific name. These were collections of colors used to decorate skin, like clothes.

Max Factor

Max Factor created make-up for Hollywood stars starting in 1909; he followed the evolution of filmmaking techniques, particularly in terms of film sensitivity and lighting effects. In 1930, it was known around the world as the "make-up of the stars" and what woman didn't dream of becoming one herself? The company is now owned by Procter and Gamble.

Guerlain

Initially a perfume-maker, Guerlain opened a beauty parlor in 1938 on the Champs Elysées after 110 years as a successful business providing scents to aristocratic clients around the world. Beauty treatments were the first products, followed with Terracotta bronze foundation in 1984.

Lancaster

Created in 1946 and initially based in Monaco (it even had a Ligne Princière, or princely line), the company was purchased in 1990 by the German group Benckiser, which further developed the company's "high-tech" character.

Lancôme
Created in the 1930s by
François Coty, Lancôme is today,
like Helena Rubenstein,
one of the "selective market"
brands of the Oréal company,
which began with hair dyes.

Estée Lauder
This company appeared after
World War II, but soon became the
world's fifth leading cosmetics
and perfume firm, with numerous
beauty treatment products
and specialized beauty care lines.

Revlon
Revlon began with fingernails in
1932, then matched lipsticks to their
polishes—in other words, the
opposite of the traditional cosmetics
company. Nonetheless, Revlon is
the seventh largest cosmetics firm.

Helena Rubinstein
This company had an unusual
development, opening shops in
Poland and Australia, before
London, Paris and New York.
Rubinstein created the first
waterproof mascara.

Shiseido
This group, which began as a
pharmacy in the late nineteenth
century, is a great ambassador
for Western culture and art in Japan,
while exporting a traditional
cosmetic culture toward the West.
Serge Lutens, who worked at Dior,
is the artistic director for both
Europe and Japan.

In addition to these major names, a
few "newcomers" have appeared;
they offer beauty products and
"studio" professional skin care to
everyone:

Shu Uemura, a pioneer in this field
which opened in 1983 in Japan;
the company opened shop in Paris
three years later.

Mac, created in 1985, has clients
such as Catherine Deneuve and
Vanessa Paradis.

Make-Up For Ever, founded by
Dany Sanz, is now on sale at
Galeries Lafayette in Paris.

By Terry, or Terry de Gunzburg.
After working ten years with Carita
and fourteen with Saint Laurent,
she pampers his clients in the
Galerie Véro-Dodat shop with a color
library, laboratory and testing rooms,
for made-to-measure cosmetics.

The books
are listed
in their
order of
appearance
in the text

Ovid, *Cosmetics*, volume III; *The Art of Love*, book III; *Complete works*

Baudelaire, *Éloge du maquillage*, in *Le Peintre de la vie moderne*, 1863, *Œuvres complètes*, Gallimard, 1961

C. Levi-Strauss, *Tristes Tropiques*, Plon, 1955; *Le Dédoublement et la représentation dans les arts de l'Asie et de l'Amérique*, in *Renaissance*, magazine of the Free School, New York, 1944–1945

France Borel, *Le Vêtement incarné*, Calmann-Lévy, 1992

P. Guth, in *Dictionnaire des produits de beauté et de cosmétologie*, Éditions 26, 1968

J. Pinset et Y. Deslandres, *Histoire des soins de beauté*, Que sais-je?, PUF, 1960

Martial, Épigramme 55, in *Gelliam*, book III, in *Toutes les épigrammes en latin et en français*, Paris, 1842–1843

Tertulliean, *Traité sur la toilette des femmes, Traité contre les spectacles*, translated by Père Matthieu Caubère, 1733

R. Cerbelaud, *Æsculape*, January 1935

A. Paul Long, *Le Miracle libéral* or *Lola Montès, ballade bavaroise*, 1847

Edgar Morin, *les Stars*, Seuil, 1957

L. -C. de Caraccioli, *Dictionnaire critique, pittoresque et sentencieux, propre à faire connaître les usages du siècle, ainsi que ses bizarreries*, Lyon, B. Duplain, 1768

E. de Goncourt, *Outamaro, le peintre des maisons vertes, l'art japonais au XVIIIe*; E. and J. de Goncourt, *La Femme au XVIIIe siècle*, 1862

Sonnini de Manoncourt, Charles-Nicolas-Sigisbert, *Voyage dans la Haute et la Basse Égypte*, Paris, F. Buisson, year VII

La Célestine, attributed to Fernando de Rojas, 1499, Aubier, 1992.

Ch. Desroches-Noblecourt, *Fards et parures au temps des pharaons*; recipe on papyrus Edwin Smith (XXI,9-XX,10); *L'Amour de l'art* no. 49-50-51, 1950–1951

Kalidasa, *le Nuage messager, les Saisons*, translated by R-H Assier de Pompigne, Paris, 1938

Homer, *Iliad*, verse XIV, ca 170–177, cited by M. Detienne, *Les Jardins d'Adonis, la mythologie des aromates en Grèce*, Gallimard, 1972

A. Cenini, *Il libro dell'Arte*, 1437, translated by Victor Mottez, one of Ingres' favorite students, 1858

G. Elgey, *La République des illusions (1945–1951)*, Fayard, 1965,1993

Théophile Gautier, *De la Mode*, (1858), Actes Sud, 1993

Y. Mishima, *Confession d'un masque*, Gallimard, 1971

B. Grillet, *Les Femmes et les Fards dans l'Antiquité grecque*, Lyon, CNRS, 1975

C. James, *Toilette d'une Romaine au temps d'Auguste et Cosmétiques d'une Parisienne au XIXe siècle*, Hachette, 3rd ed. 1879

Montaigne, *Essais*, book I, chap. XIV, Pléiade, Gallimard, 1962

Johannès Gros, *Une courtisane romantique*, Marie Duplessis, Paris, 1929

E. Rimmel, *The Book of Perfumes*, London, 1865; in French, Paris, 1867

Mémoires de la baronne d'Oberkirch sur la cour de Louis XVI et la société française avant 1789, Mercure de France, 1989

Balzac, *Petit Dictionnaire critique et anecdotique des Enseignes de Paris, par un batteur de pavé*, 1826, printed by Balzac

Comte de Vaublanc, *Mémoires*, 1782

Barbier, *Chroniques de la Régence et du règne de Louis XV*, Paris, 1857

Lesley Blanch, *Pierre Loti*, Seghers, 1986

Lola Montès, *L'Art de la beauté*, or *Secrets de la toilette des dames*, 1858

E. Arden, Company brochure, 1935

Dupetit-Thouars, *Relation du voyage autour du monde sur la frégate la Vénus*, Paris, 1840–1864

M. Mitchell, *Gone With the Wind*, 1936

Ali-Akbar Mazahéri, *La vie quotidienne des Musulmans au Moyen Âge* (Xe-XIIIe siècles) Hachette, 1951

Scarron, *Epître à Mme d'Hautefort*, in *Poésies diverses*, Paris, Librairie Marcel Didier, 1947

Lectures pour tous, Hachette, 3e trim. 1900

J. Soustelle, *La vie quotidienne des Aztèques*, Hachette, 1955

J. Haafner, *Voyages dans la péninsule occidentale de l'Inde et dans l'ile de Ceilan*, translated into French from Dutch by Mr. Jansen, Paris, Arthus-Bertrand, 1811

Jean-Luc Bonniol, *Beauté et couleur de la peau*, in *Communications* no. 60, Seuil, 1995

La Fontaine, *La Mouche et la Fourmi*, 3rd fable in book IV, dedicated to Mlle de Sévigné, 1668

Racine, *Athalie*, act II, scene 5

A. Paré, *Œuvres complètes*, édition de 1585

M. Berthelot (ed.), *Grande Encyclopédie*, published from 1885 to 1900

Louis-Sébastien Mercier, *Tableau de Paris*, Slatkine, 1979

Jacques Serena, *Rimmel*, (commissioned by Jean-Louis Martinelli for the Théâtre National de Strasbourg), Minuit, 1988

A. Caron, *La Toilette des dames*, Au Grand Buffon, Librairie de A.G. Debray, 1806

Les Secrets du seigneur Alexis piémontois, edited and complemented by an infinity of rare rares secrets, Book 6: Recpies of Various Authors, In Rouen with Pierre Amiot, 1691

Lane, Edward William, *An Account of the Manners and Customs of the Modern Egyptians*, written in Egypt during the years 1833–1834, partly from notes made during a former visit to that country in the years 1825–1828, London, 1860

Choderlos de Laclos, *Des femmes et de leur éducation*, 1783, in *Œuvres complètes*, Pléiade, Gallimard, 1979

Marie-Claude Phan et Jean-Louis Flandrin, *Les Métamorphoses de la beauté féminine*, in *L'Histoire* n°68, juin 1984

G.-L. Pringué, *30 ans de dîners en ville*, éd. revue *Adam*, 1948

Mme Cocheris, *Les Parures primitives*, Jouvet et Cie, 1914

P. Labat, *Voyage aux Caraïbes en 1700*, cited in *Traverses* no. 7, February 1977, CCI/Minuit

Simone de Beauvoir, *La Force de l'âge*, Gallimard, 1960

A. Franklin, *La Vie privée d'autrefois. Arts et Métiers, Modes, Mœurs, Usages des Parisiens du XIIe au XVIIIe siècle*, Paris, numerous volumes, 1887 for *Les soins de toilette*.

Robert Van Gulik, *La vie sexuelle dans la Chine ancienne*, Gallimard, 1971

Concernant Henri III, cf. Agrippa d'Aubigné, *Les Tragiques*, Book II, Princes, H. Champion, 1995

E.-P. Rodocanachi, *Tolla la courtisane, esquisse de la vie privée à Rome en l'an du jubilé 1700*, Paris, E. Flammarion, 1897

Marcel Mauss, *Manuel d'ethnographie* (1947), Petite Bibliothèque Payot, 1967

Dominique Veillon, *La Mode sous l'occupation, débrouillardise et coquetterie dans la France en guerre, 1939–1945*, Payot, 1990

Diderot, *Œuvres esthétiques*, Garnier, 1959

Giovanni Marinello, *Gli ornamente delle donne*, Venetia, G. Valgrisi, 1574

Christian Dior, Jacqueline Capelle de Menou, *Propos sur la mode*, in *Civilisation française*, newsletter for alumni and friends of the Cours de civilisation française, held at the Sorbonne, 1955.

Photographic credits

1 Parfums Christian Dior/photo: Tyen
2 Marc Walter/Parfums Christian Dior
5 Tyen/Parfums Christian Dior
7 By Terry/photo: P. Knaup et coll. part./photo: P. Louis
8 photo: P. Louis
9 Musée des Beaux Arts d'Angers
10 Magnum Photos/E. Arnold
11 Photo: R. Voinquel © Ministère de la Culture-France
12–13 left: Bildarchiv, Munich and private coll./photo: P. Louis
14 Photo: R. Parry © Ministère de la Culture-France
15 private coll./photo: P. Louis; top: Shu Uemura
16 Magnum Photos/B. Barbey
17 Noriaki Yokosuka
18 Guerlain
19 Guerlain and Walter coll.
20 Lauros-Giraudon/Musée de l'Annonciade
21 Photo: R. Corbeau © Ministère de la Culture-France
22 private coll./photo: P. Louis
23 Arqué coll.
24 Shiseido
25 Walter coll.
26 Photo F. Kollar © Ministère de la Culture-France
27 Photo: studio Harcourt © Ministère de la Culture-France
28 Walter coll./photo: Simon/Paris Match
29 top: private coll./photo: P. Louis; bottom: Lancôme
30 Chanel
31 Photo: J.-H. Lartigue © Ministère de la Culture-France
32–33 coll. Walter
34 Magnum Photos/Lessing
35 Musée des Beaux Arts de Lyon/photo: studio Basset
36 Rue des Archives/Everett
37 private coll./photo: P. Louis
38 Make Up For Ever
39 Walter coll.
40 Association Willy Maywald/Adagp Paris 2000
41 Archives Parfums Dior and private coll./photo: P. Louis
42–43 Marc Walter/Dior
44 Make Up For Ever
45 Marc Walter/Dior
47 Walter coll.
49 London National Gallery
50 Scala Group, Firenze
51 Walter coll.
52 Magnum Photos/Lessing
53 R. M. N./Louvre/photo: G. Blot

54 Rue des Archives and archives Piver
55 Musée du Louvre/photo: P. Louis
56 Lauros-Giraudon/Musée des Beaux Arts de Rouen
57 Bourjois
58 Château de Versailles/photo: P. Louis and Fragonard archives/photo: J.P. Dieterlen
59 Magnum Photos/Lessing
60 Lancôme and private coll./photo: P. Louis
61 Bourjois
62 private coll./photo: P. Louis
63 Magnum Photos/M. Parr
64–65 Magnum Photos/M. Franck
66 Bourjois and U.C.A.D./Musée de la Publicité
67 Archives Parfums Dior
69 R.M.N./Louvre/photo: G. Blot
70 Photo: studio Harcourt © Ministère de la Culture-France
71 Walter coll.
72 Magnum Photos/Lessing
73 Thèbes/photo: J.-P. Galerneau
74–75 Magnum Photos/Lessing
76 U.C.A.D./Musée des Arts Décoratifs/photo: Marc Walter
77 R.M.N./Louvre/photo: H. Lewandowski and U.C.A.D./Musée des Arts Décoratifs/photo: Marc Walter
78 Walter coll.
79 Musée du Louvre/photo: J.-P. Galerneau
80 Piver archives
81 Musée Marmottan/photo: Tierry Mille
82 R.M.N./Louvre/photo: Arnaudet and Blot
83 Marc Walter/Malmaison
84 Shiseido and Photo: F. Kollar © Ministère de la Culture-France
85 U.C.A.D./Musée de la Publicité
86 left : private coll./photo: P. Louis; center: Guerlain; top: Patrimoine Lanvin
87 private coll./photo: P. Louis
88 By Terry/photo: P. Knaup (top) and Parfums Dior/photo: Tyen
89 Parfums Christian Dior/photo: Tyen
90 Barry Elkis/styling: Belinda Van Santen
91 Magnum Photos/Abbas and Guerlain
93 private coll./photo: P. Louis and Rue des Archives
95 R.M.N./Orsay/photo: Jean
96 Photo: R. Voinquel © Ministère de la Culture-France

97 Magnum Photos/Lessing
98 Photo: studio Harcourt © Ministère de la Culture-France
99 Photo: R. Corbeau © Ministère de la Culture-France
100 Shiseido
101 Fotogram Stone/Hulton Deutsch Collection
102 Walter coll.
103 Artephot/Artothek
104 Photo: studio Harcourt © Ministère de la Culture-France
105 Rue des Archives
106 Archives Dior/René Gruau
107 Australian National Gallery/photo: Lewis
108 Photo: T. Le Prat © Ministère de la Culture-France
109–110 private coll./photo: P. Louis
111 Musée du Caire/photo: J.-P. Galerneau
112 Rue des Archives/Everett
113–114 Walter coll.
115 top: photo: J.-H. Lartigue © Ministère de la Culture-France; center: Parfums Christian Dior/photo: Tyen; bottom: Lancôme
116 Magnum Photos/E. Arnold
117 Magnum Photos/R. Burri
118 private coll./photo: P. Louis
119 Magnum Photos/B. Glinn
120 Archives Parfums Christian Dior
121 By Terry/photo: P. Knaup
122 Archives Parfums Christian Dior
123 Marc Walter/Dior
125 Photo: R. Voinquel © Ministère de la Culture-France
126 Guerlain
127 Parfums Christian Dior/photo: Tyen
128 Guerlain
129 private coll./photo: P. Louis
130 R.M.N./Orsay/photo: G. Blot
131 private coll./photo: P. Louis and By Terry/photo: P. Knaup
132–133 Magnum Photos/Pinkhassov
134 U.C.A.D./Musée de la Publicité
135 Bibliothèque Forney/René Gruau
136 Shu Uemura and private coll./photo: P. Louis
137 Photo: J.-H. Lartigue/ © Ministère de la Culture-France
138 R.M.N./Orsay/photo: J. Schormans

139 Magnum Photos/Lessing and Turin Museum/photo: J.-P. Galerneau
140 R.M.N./Guimet/photo: P. Willi
141 photo: J.-H. Lartigue © Ministère de la Culture-France
142 Magnum Photos/Abbas
143 Norman Rockwell Museum/Stockbridge
144 Photo: J.-H. Lartigue © Ministère de la Culture-France
145 private coll./photo: P. Louis
146 J.-M. Tardi
147 Marc Walter
148 Estée Lauder and Marc Walter
149 Shu Uemura
150–151 Marc Walter
153 Peter Knaup/By Terry
154 Parfums Christian Dior archives
155 Parfums Christian Dior/photo: Tyen
156 Lancôme and Estée Lauder
157 Lancaster/photo: P. Demarchelier
159 Shiseido Beauté
160 Norman Parkinson
161 Magnum/P. Halsman
162 U.C.A.D./Musée des Arts Décoratifs/photo: Marc Walter and private coll./photo: P. Louis
163 Dagli Orti, Paris/private coll.
164-167 private coll./photo: P. Louis
168 Lauros-Giraudon
169 Walter coll.
170 Parfums Christian Dior/photo: Tyen
171 Dior archives/René Gruau
172–173 Parfums Christian Dior/photo: Tyen
174 Magnum Photos/B. Barbey
175 Bourjois
176 Cosmos/Woodfin Camp/Seitelman
177 Magnum Photos/Pinkhassov
178 Magnum Photos/Rio Branco
179 Dior Couture archives/photo: Doucet
180 Photo : J.-H. Lartigue © Ministère de la Culture-France
181 Parfums Christian Dior/photo: Tyen
182 Paul Outerbridge (top) and private coll./photo: P. Louis
183 private coll./photo: P. Louis
184–185 Parfums Christian Dior/photo: Tyen